Let us be the first to discern what [the modern person] is saying. He [she] is thirsting for God. "The aggrandized body is waiting for the supplementation of the soul," wrote Henri Bergson, "and . . . mechanicalism requires a mysticism."

Paul Tournier
The Whole Person in a Broken World

IN THE
LAND OF THE
LIVING

Karin Granberg-Michaelson

ZONDERVAN BOOKS
Zondervan Publishing House
Grand Rapids, Michigan

THIS IS A ZONDERVAN BOOK
Published by Zondervan Publishing House
1415 Lake Drive S.E.
Grand Rapids, Michigan 49506

IN THE LAND OF THE LIVING
© 1984 by The Zondervan Corporation
Grand Rapids, Michigan

Library of Congress Cataloging in Publication Data

Granberg-Michaelson, Karin.
    In the land of the living.

    Bibliography: p.
    1. Holistic medicine.   2. Spiritual healing.   I. Title.
R723.G7   1984   615.8′52   83-27437
ISBN 0-310-27491-5

Book Designer: Kim Koning
Copy Editor: Penelope J. Stokes

Printed in the United States of America

84 85 86 87 88 / 10 9 8 7 6 5 4 3 2 1

To my father and mother,
my partner Wesley,
our son JonKrister,
and our daughter Karis Rose

Contents

Introduction

It's supposed to be a professional secret, but I'll tell you anyway. We doctors do nothing. We only help and encourage the doctor within.

Albert Schweitzer

We all want to be well. Yet, why one person is healthy and vigorous while another is weak and vulnerable to every stress is a mystery. In recent years, however, much has been discovered about the connections between life events, feelings, and illness. More people are becoming aware that emotions have power to influence health or illness.

New approaches to health care are lively news to an eager constituency. Many denominational magazines have featured articles on the relationship between faith and health. The holistic health care boom has made the covers of *Time* and *Newsweek*. Public interest is strong.

Although the media have picked up on the secular holistic health care explosion emerging out of California, less is known about whole person health care which springs out of the church's life.

Most of us are out of the habit of associating health care with the church. In fact, in some circles, religious practice and conviction are more commonly associated with neurosis than with health. Historically, however, the church is where health care began. Hospitals trace their roots to the church, and mission hospitals located all over the world testify that in the recent past, the church had a clear sense of its healing mission.

Convinced by the theory of whole-person health care, I came to experience its daily practice, not as an abstract concept, but as a personal reality. Several years ago, Dr. Janelle Goetcheus and I were brought together as we discovered a common call to provide whole-person health care in the heart of Washington, D.C. Others joined this dream, and Columbia Road Health Services was born.

This book is intended to be useful at many levels—by offering an introduction to the theology and practice of whole-person health care, by serving as a self-help resource for deeper appreciation of what constitutes wellness and moves a person toward wholeness, and by providing models to excite local churches to discover their own possibilities for developing a whole-person health care system. The appendix offers materials used by whole-person health care centers.

The effect of a person's religious faith, or the lack of it, on one's health is tremendously significant—both positive, life-enhancing faith, and debilitating, punitive religious influences. Whether we say "yes" or "no" to what life sends our way has tremendous implications for our general health.

It would be a mistake to view whole person health care as more than it is—a rather obvious linking of things that belong together, shedding light on what had been previously compartmentalized. The concept is as straightforward as this simple statement: the whole is greater than the sum of its parts.

In whole-person health care we can find new resources for health and wholeness. In any discussion of illness it is easy to create more problems than originally existed. Guilt is readily produced in those whose health is troubled and whose faith is not curative. It is not my purpose in this book to burden those who seek better health with questions about the quality of their Christian faith, but rather to offer new ways of approaching the questions of faith and health, ways that may prove useful in the search for better health and better quality life.

My first significant encounter with sickness, hospitalization, and death occurred when I was thirteen. My grandfather, who was very special to me, became ill and died in the hospital within the following two weeks. During one of the last conversations I had with my grandfather at his hospital bedside, I urged him to try to recover; I tried to bargain with him by reminding him of his prized rose garden at home. His response was that he was too tired and that the flowers would go on without him. He was ready, even eager, to let go of his life and move on to his heavenly home.

Looking back at this encounter, I realize that I learned at thirteen that we all have some measure of power and influence over our health. Like most people, I regarded the doctors I saw as magicians who dispensed the right medications and produced saving results; I credited them with wisdom and discernment far exceeding their scientific knowledge. Yet our own attitudes help to determine how long we will live, what diseases we will suffer, and how we may journey toward recovery or find wholeness even in the midst of terminal illness.

And, like most people, I have often found it easier to consult with doctors than to look for unresolved feelings or a spiritual emptiness that might help to explain my physical symptoms. By saying this, I don't mean to imply that our physical make-up plays no part in our health. There can be a predisposition for a particular set of physical problems. For example, I am troubled by occasional asthma and allergies, as are several members of my family. But I have learned that sometimes I am able to reduce the severity of an asthma attack by taking time to think about current pressures and feelings. While this discipline may strike some as tedious or self-absorbed, for me and many others this relationship between stress and illness is a key to improved health.

Paul Tournier's medical experience has convinced him that a spiritual unrest underlies almost every chronic and acute illness. When this unrest reaches great enough proportions, it throws the body's systems out of balance. Tournier encourages his patients to probe deeply into the feelings that accompany their physical or emotional illness. They often discover a need to make restitution to someone, perhaps a parent or spouse. When patients pursue the roots of their illness and mend broken relationships, their balance is restored. Then, and only then, a measure of healing takes place. In most cases, of course, healing is a long process. But it is often set in motion when people face the alienation and sin that precipitated the illness.

My own study of the psychology of religion has made me aware of the spiritual roots of illness in my own life. Illness often has its roots in feelings of guilt and the need to be reconciled. For the sake of our health we must learn to listen to our conscience and recognize more clearly the pangs of *true* guilt that demand restitution.

To do this, it is especially important that we learn to sense the difference between true and false guilt. Tournier suggests that true guilt comes from within the quietness of our own heart. The things for which God reproaches us are usually quite different from the things for which others reproach us. Too often we want to turn away—to deaden the voice which demands a scrupulous integrity before God. But ignoring the pangs of authentic guilt can prove costly to the body.

If my body hurts, I can learn to allow the pain to instruct me. When I am wheezing with asthma, I can ask, "What is sitting so heavily on my chest?" If I feel free to search my heart for something that may be amiss in my relationship to God, to those in my family, or to myself, then I may find release. Feelings and thoughts may seem painful and threatening, but we must not allow our bodies to pay for them—rather, we must bring them into the light to be seen, understood and healed.

Holistic health care can be the most comprehensive and effective care a person can receive. Being seen as a whole person, gaining insight into one's attitudes and behavior are important factors in the healing process. We need an environment where all the major influences in our lives can be examined simultaneously and a comprehensive treatment plan devised. Perhaps the chief benefit of whole person medical practice is the corporate wisdom of the professional team. What one member perceives can be checked with the others. What one member overlooks, another may detect. We are complex beings, and our health care system should be built around this conviction.

Whole person health care is not a panacea for a broken world. It will not produce a cure where cure is not possible. But it may help us to see ourselves more as Scripture does, and as God does—whole people who need to strive toward harmony with ourselves, God, and others.

1 | In the Land of the Living: Helene's Story

"I am still confident of this: I will see the goodness of the Lord in the land of the living."

Psalm 27:13 NIV

Born into a conservative Christian home in a rural community, Helene was the oldest of five children. Her early life was shaped by strict adherence to the work ethic for her family and church, and she grew up believing that striving to do and be the best was what God required of her. It was also what pleased those around her.

When Helene was seventeen, she experienced a severe and abrupt loss. One day, her mother became critically ill. Helene was the only child at home, and her father sent her to call the doctor. Just as Helene left the room to make the call her mother died. Helene's father would not let her back into her mother's room, and Helene became very upset when her next sight of her mother was in a coffin. Helene feared that her mother might be suffocating.

Eventually, Helene swallowed her grief and tried to resume her life. Shortly after her mother's death, Helene's father remarried. After this, Helene left home and began nurse's training.

Helene became an R.N. and accepted a position at a mission hospital on an Indian reservation. Then, Helene had what she later realized was a near-death experience.

She was home with her family for a visit and vacation, and had an accident while water skiing. By the time her family had transported her to a nearby hospital, she had no measurable blood pressure and no pulses. She was covered with hives the size of dinner plates and shivering with a body temperature of 93 degrees. Her color was bluish purple. Listening to those around her, Helene knew she was dying.

Meanwhile Helene was conscious in "another space" where she was walking down the road with a friend. Without exchanging words, she knew it was Jesus and that they were on their way to heaven. She was filled with a calm, peaceful feeling. Then she heard a nurse's voice reporting her blood pressure. And at that point the Lord silently turned around with Helene and walked back toward earth.

Helene lived, but she did not recover. Instead she became a victim of constant pain and chronic illness. She spent her days visiting doctors and hospitals trying to diagnose her mysterious disease and to find the right medication to relieve her pain.

All the elaborate tests produced negative results until finally an immunologist discovered that Helene had a rare disease of the immune system—an incurable illness, with no adequate medication to control the pain. Helene became a prisoner of her bedroom, often too weak to lift her head from her pillow. And, as a final indignity, she had become allergic both to the sun's rays and to all forms of cold—the weather, cold beverages, even cold water. Her muscles throbbed and she coughed incessantly. All the pleasures of her life vanished.

One of the saving graces of Helene's situation was that she was a member of a Christian fellowship and she lived with members of her community who prayed with her and cared for all her physical needs during her years of illness. But even this support was inadequate against the pain Helene was experiencing.

The strange circumstances that had cast her into a life of sickness and pain instead of her former health and competence were propelling Helene into a new world of inner turmoil and fear. Did she really have a terminal disease, or was she imagining her pain? Would she spend the rest of her life sick and dependent? What did God want her to learn from this continuing illness?

Helene kept a journal and recorded her questions and feelings of doubt and anger toward God. All the while she wished she had died and gone to heaven in Christ's company. But she was alive—alive to another day, another month, another year of physical pain and mental anguish.

During this period of hopelessness, Helene discovered a verse from the Bible which became a motto for her. In Psalm 27:13 she glimpsed the beginning of her answer. "I would have despaired unless I had believed that I would see the goodness of the Lord in the land of the living." God seemed to have a purpose for her life which was to be fulfilled here on earth rather than through death. Helene determined to try to experience what goodness God might be offering her even in the midst of her illness and pain.

But Helene's health did not improve. Finally, her physician suggested thoracic surgery. At this point she was taking twenty to thirty pills a day to control her abnormal immunological reactions, twelve of which were for pain control. Nothing was working. The surgery would remove the ribs causing the pain, but her doctor gave her no guarantees that this high-risk procedure would lessen the pain. Helene felt desperate.

A friend in Helene's church asked whether Helene would ever consider hypnosis for pain control as an alternative to surgery. This friend referred Helene to a Christian psychologist who used what he called positive imaging with his clients.

Positive imaging is a powerful communication process which facilitates a state of deep physical relaxation and a sharp focusing of the client's mental and emotional energies along specific directed channels. As an integral part of this communication process the client's rigid ways of organizing reality are somewhat altered. Conceptual molds which have long been set are softened, allowing for change and growth.

Hypnotic suggestion is actually this process of evoking and utilizing a patient's own mental processes in ways that are outside his/her usual range of intentional or voluntary control. This psychologist believed that a person's own powerfully protective and understanding unconscious mind, where our spirit and the Spirit of God live together, allows us to experience whatever feelings, thoughts or images that are needed for the healing process.

On Helene's first visit to the psychologist, he led her through a relaxation exercise using positive imaging. This reminded Helene of being with Christ in her near-death experience and had a very calming effect. When she used the relaxation exercises her therapist taped for her, she began to notice a decrease in pain. With continuous use and therapeutic interviews her pain continued to decrease and she began to use less medication. The psychologist told her he believed that her subconscious and the Lord knew what it would take to heal her body. Helene did not believe this, but she was seeing some improvement so she continued her visits.

During this time, Helene began to see connections between the stress and tension in her life and her bodily disease. She wanted to excel and to do everything well. Part of the pain in her prolonged illness was how useless she had become. She could not imagine being of any value in her weakness.

Things became further complicated when Helene's immunologist began subtlely to question the remarkable healing effects which were occurring in Helene's counseling process. This tension between specialists created more anxiety in Helene and uncertainty of how to listen to these doctors and sort through their advice. Fortunately, her doctors were sensitive enough to Helene to realize the need for their thorough cooperation. When they resolved to work together toward Helene's health and well-being, she began to improve again.

About two months into this intensive therapy, Helene began to gain some insight about some deeply unresolved feelings about her mother's death. She began having thoughts that she might be trying to stay connected to her mother by wishing to join her through death. When others had commented on how like her mother she was, she had begun to believe that like her mother she would die young. Perhaps she was a contributor to all this illness!

Before her illness Helene had functioned as a pastoral counselor and leader in her church community. Her church was to host an annual meeting of church community leaders from various parts of the country, and Helene wanted to feel well enough to participate normally. She was furious when weakness and pain overtook her and part of her fury was the shame of appearing so weak and needy in front of all these leaders. She wanted to be a peer, not a person in real need of healing in body, mind and spirit.

Although Helene had to miss most of the meetings, she attended a worship service and requested prayer after sharing her story and her feelings of anguish. While they were praying with her, two community leaders received a sense that Helene was filled with deep self-hatred and a subconscious unwillingness to live which were contributing to her disease. Helene's close friend and pastor shared this with her and Helene became even more overwhelmed with confusion and hopelessness. After all this meaningless suffering, someone was suggesting that she was responsible for creating her illness!

After a while, Helene decided to consult with her psychologist about the community leaders' input. Much to her shock, he agreed completely and began to try to help her look at some of the facts that made these theories legitimate. Helene was horrified by what she saw in herself. She did not think of herself as someone filled with self-hatred, and she did not realize that her feelings about her mother's traumatic death could possibly be troubling her this many years later! Most of all, she could hardly believe that she, a nurse and pastoral counselor engaged in such serious Christian ministry, could fall victim to this blindness about herself and be a contributor to her disease.

The gracious understanding of members of her church enabled Helene to tolerate these painful insights and to try to work to understand herself more deeply. They encouraged her to stay involved in her pastoral work with others, because of sensitivity and insight, and believed that God was working in her and in Tom, her psychologist, to reveal the things Helene needed to know to move toward wholeness and health.

Tom encouraged Helene to "stop working so hard intellectually. Relax and trust the Holy Spirit to reveal the truth you need." In keeping with this advice, in the following sessions with her, Tom used deep relaxation and imaging techniques, along with the following story.

"Once there was a little duckling. She had no feathers to protect herself, so she was very vulnerable. Everything she encountered hurt her, even normal elements like sun and cold. In the cold, the little duck shivered and shook; in the brightness of the sun, she was burned. It even hurt her to walk among the weeds or over the stones in the everyday duck habitat.

"Then, one day, without knowing why, the duckling began to grow soft down. And soon she had a coat of protective feathers. Happily she went down to the lakeshore and joined the other ducks. She could swim and paddle and even walk without getting hurt. She could stand the cold and the sun. She could lead a normal duck life and thus was at peace."

This simple parable struck a response in Helene. By grace she developed a willing eagerness to look at the death wish in herself and to understand and be set free from it. The little duck had two choices: die for lack of protective feathering, or live, receiving the new feathers which were being provided for her. Letting go of her felt need for her mother and letting go of the sickness and pain that kept her feeling close to her mother were the only ways for Helene to accept her circumstances and move on with her own life.

Helene began to have many revelatory dreams, each

specifically connected to the issues she was grappling with. She dreamed about being a child in her mother's arms with her grip tight around her mother's neck. In her dream, she sensed that Jesus was trying to help her let go, even prying at her fingers—but she refused, crying out to her mother, "I need you so much!"

Helene began to remember her mother's death, viewing her in the casket at the funeral home and the burial service. In her mind her mother was not dead; the casket and burial were suffocating her. Inwardly, Helene was hysterical with grief over losing someone she loved and needed so much. But at the actual service she acted in the fashion of her family and tried to bury all these intense emotions with her mother's body in the dark of her unconscious.

It was Easter Sunday. Listening to the sermon, Helene felt she was ready to stop clinging to her mother and move on. She dialogued with her mom in her journal and said good-bye for the first time in seventeen years. Arriving back home, she realized that her remaining physical pain was gone. Writing these events in her journal she concluded, "It seems I'm free to live—Hallelujah!"

There was still more work to do, and Helene was ready. She continued her visits to her psychologist and the use of positive imaging as well as the keeping of a journal; but in daily ways she has experienced health and wholeness growing up inside her and strengthening her body. Helene's psychological and spiritual insights correspond to her rare disease of the immune system. The immune system is the body's protection. Could Helene, anxious to protect herself from further pain and grief, set up a war within herself and ruin her own natural protective system? Whatever the reasons, Helene, like the little duck, found herself featherless and unprotected despite intense self-protective measures. By some mysterious circumstance Helene received the gift of a different kind of feathering, totally distinct from her own attempts to control her life and protect herself. These new feathers gave true security based on a sense of peace and well-being in God's love and acceptance.

Later, Helene read an article which described how the body's immune system can sometimes overprotect itself. For example, it may see danger where there is none, reacting physiologically to this perceived danger with excessive releases of histamine, the substance which caused many of Helene's symptoms. Helene wondered if her body had received continual messages of danger because of her self-hatred and wish to die. In its effort to respond to these messages, her immune system turned against her. Had she not pursued the avenue of emotional and spiritual insight, her disease might have had more serious consequences. But when, through counseling, she began seeing and understanding what was going on beneath the surface of herself, her body responded positively to the new messages of hope and a renewed will to live. It began releasing less toxic amounts of histamine, and gradually subsided to normal levels.

In June, nine months after entering therapy, Helene visited her hometown to complete the process of letting go of her mother and her anguished past. She visited her mother's grave for the first time since her burial so many years before. She planted a crocus as a sign of her love, and wondered why this letting go had taken her so long.

Helene regretted that so many years had slipped by in the fog of unresolved grief. How could her normal grief over the loss of a person as significant as her mother have become so abnormal, with such far-reaching physical, spiritual and emotional effects? One of the keys may be the fact that in an effort to protect her, Helene's father would not let Helene go back into the bedroom and see her mother dead. By being kept out of the room and away from funeral arrangements, Helene did not come to terms with her dead parent, and through the following years continued to need her mother close at hand, even if that meant being together in illness, or ultimately being reunited through death.

When Helene returned from her trip home, she visited her immunologist who told her that blood tests showed her disease to be in remission. At last she was seeing the goodness of the Lord in the land of the living!

Helene continued to gain in health and strength, although she still found it necessary to maintain her health and well-being through the use of daily relaxation/meditation using her positive imaging tapes, walking or other physical exercise, and a conscious effort to receive her strength from God, not her own effort. This program was so vital to promoting her continuing health that she considered the specific components spiritual disciplines.

Helene eventually resumed her full work load as a pastoral counselor, youth director and ministry coordinator in her church. She was also still licensed as a registered nurse in her state. In November of 1982, she traveled to South India to share her experiences at a symposium on faith and health which took place at the Vellore Christian Medical College and Hospital.

How are we to understand what happened to Helene, and what value does her story have for us? During her recovery process, Helene occupied herself with reading and reflecting. One book in particular seemed to express her situation, *My God, My God: Answers to our Anguished*

Cries, by Ruth Vaughn. Vaughn described what she experienced:

> My entire understanding of life was founded in activity, performance and giving. My entire understanding of God was founded in service. The equation I had built my definition of life upon . . . the equation I had built my concept of God upon was: performance = goodness, non-performance = badness. And performance was intrinsically linked with health. I saw illness as bad—I was no longer worthy of life, no longer of value in God-service.

After she encountered illness and even death, she wrote:

> Now I had the freedom, courage and faith to begin to build for the second period of my life much as I built for the first: with my whole heart, creatively. My "badness" did not destroy the world of activity. My "goodness" has nothing whatever to do with performance.
>
> God did not create me to perform for Him, but He created me as His child . . . to love me, to find me "precious," to call me "honorable." I faced life with Him. He created me to be with Him. He had created me to be me. Yes, my life was starting over again—everything seemed new and different.

Ruth Vaughn's thoughts and feelings echo Helene's. Both tried to live life according to a merit system, and when struck down by illness, they concluded that they were worthless and bad. After weathering pain and illness, each gained new insight about life as a gift based on God's willing acceptance of her human condition. In time Helene, like Ruth Vaughn, began to experience a great sense of personal freedom and joy in living.

Helene's near-death encounter seemed to act as a catalyst which stimulated a number of feelings that were buried beneath the surface of her daily life. She found herself questioning her purpose in life, particularly as she did not bounce back to health, but was troubled with chronic pain and weakness. She vacillated between feeling that nothing was really wrong and being angry over her weakness; ultimately fearing that she indeed had a terminal illness and attempting to bargain with God for her life.

Despite such conflicting emotions, Helene retained a sense that somewhere in her trouble God was present—that even in the darkest moments God was with her and was working with her for her ultimate good. Such faith existing side by side with a subconscious death wish and self-hatred may reveal something of the complexity of human personality.

Helene's own interpretation of her illness was that God was using her weakness to reveal reality to her—that she was acceptable in whatever state she was in and could not earn God's favor through her former boundless energy and good works. Helene's committed relationship of faith in God and God's purposes, as well as her committed life in Christian community, gave her a powerful resource which helped her endure the hopelessness she often felt. As the illness wore on and worsened, her questions began to focus on mere survival rather than a search for understanding. At the worst, she longed for a way out.

After being in therapy for a while, Helene began to try to relax into her situation—to allow herself to be supported physically, emotionally and spiritually by those around her, to stop fighting. Her psychologist encouraged Helene to celebrate the smallest positive step forward and used positive imaging to try to alter her viewpoint. She began to utilize daily periods of rest and relaxation in order to quiet herself and center in to a peaceful state.

These times of tranquil meditation and focusing on positive imaging sped the healing process along. Once Helene recovered a will to live, she began to better understand how her former way of life had hindered her, and she learned what steps she could take to maintain her health and sense of well-being. She learned enough about herself to begin to recognize her own warning signals.

As Helene gained in strength she began to be curious about the role that prolonged emotional distress had played in the development of her illness. That question is still being answered, but she has enough information to be convinced that the emotional trauma of her mother's death, accompanied by the accumulation of normal daily stress and strain, eventually broke down her body's ability to protect her health, and disease set in. There is no question that, for Helene, learning to experience God's acceptance set her free to relax into a sense of peace and well-being which eventually translated into actual physical gains.

Helene's insights match those of Norman Cousins, author of *My Incredible Self-Cure* and *Anatomy of an Illness*. Cousins, diagnosed with a terminal illness, took the offensive and discovered several keys which eventually opened the door to health and healing in his life. Those he considers critical factors in his cure, and they further validate Helene's experience. He notes that people with a sense of purpose in life recover faster. He cites the will to live, faith, and good humor as important elements of becoming well. He also notes the importance of trust between doctor and patient, including teamwork between doctor and patient in the treatment plan. Cousins believes that patients must have a sense of responsibility for themselves, rather than constantly looking to others to solve their problems.

Of particular significance to Helene's case are Cousins' assertions that the body has the capacity to regenerate itself, and that people must be willing to try, to use whatever it takes to trigger this ability of the body to right itself. Finally, he says that positive emotions—creativity, will to live, hope, faith, and love—are not only life-giving, but have actual biochemical significance which contributes strongly to healing and a sense of well-being.

The remaining question is how Helene's story applies to church-related health care. Helene was fortunate in that, unlike most people who experience serious illness, her care became coordinated by a team of caring people, dedicated to assisting her recovery. These individuals had no formal ties, which makes their cooperation all the more noteworthy. Helene herself became the linking person who brought together the insights of her physicians, pastors, and her counseling psychologist. Because of this cooperation, Helene's body, mind and spirit began to be treated simultaneously. Had there been a holistic health care clinic available when she first became ill, her illness might have been brought under control sooner.

What happens to the rest of us during times of illness and crisis? Most of us do not have access to doctors, pastors, and counselors working as a team to promote our total well-being. All too often our care is fragmented and there is no continuity in our treatment. Each time we visit a new specialist we start over, rather than building on inter-related aspects of the illness.

The following chapters of this book will describe how such a holistic health treatment plan operates, and where this type of health care is being delivered both in the United States and overseas. We will look further at those aspects of Christian faith which seem to impact our health both for good and ill. We will also give a Biblical rationale for participation in a holistic view of persons and their health. And we will give some examples of how almost any local church and church member could become involved in health-related ministries.

Many people do not recover a measure of health as Helene did, but perhaps the drama of her story will inspire us to think openly about the parallels which we find in our own lives. Through considering her experiences we may come to a better understanding of the links between prolonged distress and illness. We may even discover new approaches toward our own journey toward wholeness.

2 | Faith and Health: Wholeness in Body, Mind, and Spirit

I do not need to stir up any religious disquietude in my patients. I know that they are full of it already and far more consciously than they admit.

Paul Tournier, The Whole Person in a Broken World

The Christian faith embodied in the local church should be our greatest resource in moving toward a sense of wholeness—but often it is not. The faith which is available to liberate seems to backfire and ensnare people in feelings of guilt and self-hatred. Although faith played a strong role in Helene's recovery process, her early experiences in the church seem in some measure responsible for her striving for perfection.

Church-related health care can focus attention on the faith dimensions of our lives. By giving people opportunity to talk about their beliefs, it can function as a corrective in certain cases where childhood faith experiences have been hurtful. Whether our faith functions as an asset or a liability to our sense of well-being and health, it almost certainly affects our health in some way.

When a pastoral counselor at a church-based holistic health center meets a client for an initial interview, clients have proved surprisingly ready to talk about their faith, whether they are practicing Christians or not. Everyone seems to know that faith is significant, but how does it affect health? The impact of faith on health cannot be verified through hard data, but faith seems to play an important role in the healing process. Conversely, lack of faith may also play a role in contributing to illness.

People have an inner understanding that there is more to life and health than scientific facts and procedures. In fact, many ultimately seem to know what is bothering them. Given a supportive, professionally skilled team such a person can make major strides toward recovery and wholeness. Albert Schweitzer called this source "the doctor within." Whether or not people acknowledge Christ, most know that the forces which shape our health are connected to something both within and beyond themselves.

Truly, as Swiss physician Paul Tournier believes, many people do carry unresolved feelings concerning significant relationships such as with their parents or spouse. These conflicting emotions, if left unresolved and unacknowledged over a period of years, prove to be emotionally debilitating, in turn producing symptoms which eventually interfere with their daily lives. Some of these symptoms express themselves emotionally through recurrent disturbing thoughts, the inability to concentrate, frequent crying or angry outbursts. Inner conflicts can also translate into bodily expressions such as sleeplessness or exhaustion, frequent severe headaches, dizziness, stomach or bowel upsets, rashes or difficulty in breathing. These and many other physical manifestations of emotional discomfort may occur when we ignore conflicts that are troubling us over a long period of time.

Through the counseling process, clients often discover more about why their body is giving them trouble. After reaching the root of their trouble—whether it is related to general guilt and anxiety, or some specific event which has not been fully understood, accepted and dealt with—many experience some relief from these physical symptoms. Even when the troubling symptoms persist, people often gain enough understanding to learn to accept and manage these symptoms without the same degree of fear and stress. Whether people are troubled by marital conflict, loss of a loved one through death or divorce, or lack of direction vocationally and spiritually, they usually experience bodily symptoms which accompany their upset thoughts and feelings. Such symptoms are natural, of course, because human beings were not created in separate compartments. The scriptures graphically illustrate bodily analogies which represent the unity of the soul and mind, particularly in the psalms of David (see Psalms 6; 31:9–17; 32; 38; 41).

Both Paul Tournier and psychologist O. H. Mowrer emphasize the centrality of acknowledgement of sin or wrongdoing to the counseling process. Acknowledging and taking responsibility for one's actions may lead to confession, even restitution, where doing so would not create an even greater injury. The receiving of forgiveness which follows is central to the healing process. Often a person cannot take these steps directly with the people involved, but the general process of taking responsibility for one's actions, confessing, and receiving forgiveness has a restorative effect. Mowrer calls this specific approach to counseling *integrity therapy*.

During my years in seminary, Tournier's writing spoke to me most clearly and personally, particularly the book *Guilt and Grace.* An evangelical Christian with a conservative theology, Tournier communicates a compassion which enables him to speak the truth in love to clients and readers. For many of us being right often seems more valuable than being understanding, but Tournier has been able to preserve a strong Christian identity, offering hard truths to people in a spirit of Christlike forgiveness.

Tournier says that the painful path of sin and humiliation opens up to the royal road of grace and freedom. This statement is a beacon of hope, leading toward an experience of God's freeing grace, allowing us to extend it to our friends and family.

Self-hatred is a dominant theme in many disorders that people suffer, as Tournier and Mowrer would attest. However, rather than attributing the destructive effects of self-hatred to unjust or false guilt—a popular explanation among certain professionals—these men share the conviction that illness often develops because we are not living up to our consciences. We reproach ourselves and make ourselves sick over things that do not ultimately matter, while we often miss areas, attitudes, and actions which are wrong and must be made right.

Both as a client and as a counselor I have found that we often reproach ourselves for issues of less consequence than our unforgiveness toward those who have injured us. Holding a grudge against someone who has wronged us may produce far more serious physical and emotional discomfort than a clearly disobedient action for which one has sincerely repented.

One couple struggled with bitterness and unforgiveness. The wife had committed adultery during a time when her husband was experiencing personal illness. A Christian, she became convicted of her sin, confessed it to her husband, and tried to make amends and go forward with her husband. Although he said he had forgiven her for this hurtful breach of trust, he unconsciously but repeatedly reproached her. He also evidenced a complete lack of trust in her, all the while insisting that he loved her and that she was to blame for the strained communication between them. Tragically, he never received insight into the lack of forgiveness which controlled all his actions and attitudes toward her since she had failed him through adultery.

In time she grew tired of his attacks and lack of confidence in her. After repeated efforts to get him to build a new life together through marriage counseling, she separated from him. She felt that there was no hope as long as he failed to realize that he had never been able to forgive her, and that his lack of forgiveness, not her adultery, was slowly poisoning their entire relationship. The headaches, stomach pains, weakness, and panicky feelings (physical symptoms) which motivated her to seek professional help were greatly improved by her confession in counseling of her wrong attitudes and actions.

Recognition of sinful actions and attitudes needs to be balanced with compassion and understanding. We base this compassion not on some prideful insistence that we are okay as we are, but on God's gracious acceptance of us in our sinful condition. We do not need to justify ourselves or attempt to placate our consciences; rather, we need to heed the messages of a sensitive conscience. Along with St. Paul, we need to acknowledge that our good intentions are not strong enough to keep us in the right—that, like my client, we are dependent on the grace of God which allows us to have compassion on ourselves and others. This fundamental freedom makes a movement toward wholeness possible, despite whatever symptoms still trouble us.

Psychologist Carl Jung offers some stimulating ideas on faith and health. Although Jung was not an orthodox evangelical in his religious thinking, he believed that spiritual issues were at the heart of the majority of his clients' troubles. He had the notion that we all must learn to accept our sinful natures, our "shadow." Jung was convinced that in doing so, we would discover buried treasure in ourselves—vast resources for creative good. He believed that the shadow needs our full acceptance before we can become liberated from its negative effects.

Jung believed that in some way God was a part of this process of self-acceptance. Above the study door where he met with clients was the motto, "Invited or uninvited, God is present here." Thus he kept the spritual dimensions of illness ever present in the counseling process.

These teachers have recognized through common experiences in their own lives and those of their clients—both in counseling and medical practice—that faith does contribute not only to a person's world view but to his total health.

A young woman suffering from severe asthma and sporadic attacks of weakness, dizziness, and occasional fainting had visited many doctors about her persistent condition, but without result. She heard about the holistic approach from a friend and decided to visit our health center. When a physical examination, including numerous types of tests, revealed no physical origin for her symptoms, the physician recommended she pursue counseling. The young woman agreed, even though she was convinced that the cause of her problems was physical. She was sure the problem would disappear once the right combination of tests and medication was found.

When a brain scan ruled out the possibility of a tumor, which could have explained her symptoms, all her excuses were used up. As counseling proceeded, it became clear that a traumatic event during college as well as several difficult experiences during her childhood had produced an overload of fear and anxiety. In addition she was deeply involved with a non-Christian boyfriend and had many unresolved feelings about how her Christian faith related to that relationship. Although a bright, capable person involved in a demanding job which she usually handled very ably, she continually retreated to her parents in times of stress.

Throughout counseling she remained hopeful that something physical was causing all her troubles. It seemed too frightening for her to believe that any one of the pressures she was feeling could have been responsible for her anxiety attacks. Gradually, she realized that some basic unresolved issues in her life had tremendous power over her. She came to see that she had been nearly incapacitated by fear and exhaustion. Whenever she was highly anxious, she would be prone to onslaughts of asthma, dizziness or weakness.

Although it took time and perseverance, this young woman learned that she could search for and recognize what was troubling her. She even learned to dispel some of the physical symptoms. By beginning to write in a journal about her family, her spiritual conflicts, and her specific fears, she discovered many of the causes of her physical distress. After several counseling sessions, this young woman gained lasting insights and relative freedom from her troublesome symptoms.

The holistic approach to health problems places much of the responsibility for wellness on the client. Many people have a natural resistance to such responsibility, expecting the doctor to "know it all" and "do it all" for them. Most of us have given the doctor tremendous and often inappropriate power over our lives, not realizing that the doctor is human, limited, and often perplexed about how to proceed with our treatment. We fear the realization that the potential source of good health may lie within us, and that a doctor's role is more appropriately to help us touch our inner wellspring of wholeness.

Another woman who sought out the holistic health center did so because of a severe lack of energy. She was convinced that she was suffering from anemia. Although she had only a part-time job, she was exhausted at the end of every work day.

A thorough physical examination revealed no physical cause for her complaint. When counseling was recommended, she told the counselor that she was involved in an extra-marital sexual relationship. Consequently, she felt torn by love for her boyfriend and unhappy with what she saw as sinfulness in herself.

Over a period of several months, she came to grips with the fact that not living up to her own standards was depressing her by means of paralyzing exhaustion. As she examined her feelings and behavior, she made several changes in her lifestyle, and her energy gradually began to return. By learning to pay attention to her body, feelings, and spiritual sensitivity her life became more whole and her health gradually improved.

Most of us find it less threatening to assume rational, physical explanations for the various illnesses which plague us than to believe that our sickness is integrally related to our spiritual and emotional state. Yet a whole range of illnesses have psychosomatic, or body-soul roots. One of the gifts of modern psychology to the church is that it has shed light on this range of illnesses—illnesses which can be healed if we pay attention to their roots. Migraine headaches, asthma, arthritis, ulcers and colitis all relate to a person's psychological and spiritual condition.

Certain types of cancer have recently been shown to have psychosomatic roots. While many of us find this hard to accept, we need to do more thinking about what makes us sick and keeps us sick.

The simple expression, "I feel sick" reveals the close connection in our thinking between feelings and health. Yet a major block to healing is that we often do not know what we feel, and so we never recognize what our feelings are telling us about our health.

The church has much to learn here. Often, in the company of Christians, people feel compelled to keep the range of their feelings from coming to light. If the church wants to promote healing that endures, it must encourage people to share their true feelings—and what better place is there for openness than in the context of Christ's healing grace and compassion?

Physical and emotional health bears signs of the stresses and strains that we experience in our inner selves; we all reveal ourselves this way. Yet any simplistic equation between our spiritual condition and subsequent illness may overlook the tragic flaw in the fiber of the fallen nature. If the sins of the parents will be visited upon the coming generations, we cannot bear total responsibility for all illnesses which befall us. Disease may be handed down genetically; we may be predisposed to certain psychological weaknesses or physiological vulnerabilities.

As Paul Tournier says, no one is exempt from suffering:

There is not life which, from birth, does not already have to carry the weight of hereditary weaknesses, which does not suffer emotional shocks in childhood, which does not suffer daily injustices, hinderances, injuries, and disappointments. To all this pain must be added, infirmity, material difficulties, bereavement, old age, worry about loved ones, and accidents. In the lives of even the most privileged there is something that is hard to accept.

Some people have, happily, inherited more perfect bodies and stronger minds than others. That inequity must ultimately be left to God's providence and care. We did not design ourselves. On the other hand, no one is perfect. When I come upon people who seem to be paragons of physical and emotional health, I often sense that they, too, have weaknesses. They have simply learned to handle their defenses better and have sometimes become more successful at repressing their true feelings.

Some individuals are genuinely more thick-skinned than others. In like manner, some are born thin-skinned. Such individuals are like the aspen trees, trembling at the slightest wind that stirs. They are vulnerable to all the stresses and strains of living; like highly-tuned instruments, they absorb every vibration. Naturally, their health is more affected by those tensions which, at least superficially do not seem to register on those with a harder shell.

As some have discovered, breaking with one's traditions or peer group can also contribute to ill health. Psychologist Karen Horney suggests that a price is paid by each person who dares to be different from the accepted norms of society. Isaiah portrays the Messiah as paying the price in his own body for the sufferings of sinful humanity; perhaps physical and psychological wear and tear are a liability of being prophetic.

I do not want to make the problem of health too simple, denying the inherent mystery of our lives. We must remember the image of the suffering servant. That is the kind of voluntary suffering the church as Christ's body sometimes experiences in giving ourselves to heal the wounds of the world.

We must strike a balance: although we know that we cannot control our health, it is vitally important to take responsibility for those aspects of health which are ours to determine. We can no longer afford to live under the illusion that body and soul have no effect on each other. We must look for ways to come to terms with the physical and emotional effects of our inner alienation from God and neighbor.

We know that the root of human misery is sin. Our health, too, reflects this spiritual condition. We are in constant need of a profound reconciliation with God and God's will for us, for such a reconciliation promotes wholeness.

3 | What Is Holistic Health Care?

Four out of five times, I'd find out what was wrong sooner if I started by examining the patient's home life, his job and his bank account instead of his heart, his digestive system and his kidneys.

Dr. Robert M. Cunningham, Jr., of the Mayo Clinic

Holistic or whole-person care is health care that attempts to treat the person as a unity of body, mind and spirit. It assumes that health is a composite result of emotions and spiritual orientation as well as physical condition. This concept is expressed in the Old Testament unity between body and spirit prior to the introduction of Greek dualism.

In practical terms, whole-person care treats each person's illness as multi-dimensional, particularly focusing on the emotional and spiritual factors which have contributed to getting sick. It recognizes the close connection between a person's sense of well-being (or lack of it) and physical health. We have pointed out that feelings of alienation from God and significant others, anger, guilt and frustration eventually find expression in bodily and emotional health if they are not attended to. Whole-person

41

health care takes particular interest in the range of pschosomatic illnesses in which soul and body appear to be divided and working against the total health of a person.

We must remember that the division between body and soul is not part of our Christian heritage. The Hebrew understanding of persons was that they are a unity of body and soul. In our culture, however, we have accepted a dualistic view of the person and have tended to separate body from spirit. Persons cannot be successfully treated apart from this holistic approach. Holistic medicine is clearly a concept and practice whose time has come.

Because of the widespread divergence in holistic health care and practice it is important to explain that church-based holistic health care confines itself to traditional medical practice with a special emphasis on the emotional, spiritual and nutritional factors in illness. A primary motivation is to return health care to the domain of the church. Secular expressions of holistic health care, on the other hand, often include Eastern religious practice and paramedical approaches to healing such as yoga, herbal remedies or megadoses of vitamins.

A primary commitment of Christians involved in whole-person health care, however, is to return health care to the domain of the church. Following is a list of general holistic health principles, most of which correspond to those practiced within church-related health programs. These summary concepts further illustrate what makes holistic health care unique.

A person is more than the sum total of the parts. It is important to consider the body/mind/spirit as inseparable entities.

High-level wellness and health are the basic thrust, not disease.

People are *clients* not patients. The client assumes responsibility in negotiating for his/her care routine.

The concept is self-care, self-help.

New attitudes toward birth, health, life, illness, and death are adopted.

Stress and tension are the precursors of disease.

A practitioner of holistic health acts only as a catalyst for the client to maintain or strengthen his/her own body balance, homeostatis, or immunity, thus alleviating his/her own condition as necessary.

The methods which the practitioner uses to foster this harmony and balance are based on the belief in a higher order of consiousness.

The common thread in these principles is an openness to all aspects of human experience, responsibility-taking, and an awareness that there is a higher source than the natural order which influences a person's life and health. Compare these ideas with your own attitudes about illness and medical treatment.

The chief pioneer in the church-related holistic health movement is Granger Westberg, founder of Wholistic Health Centers, Inc. (WHC, Inc.), the spawning institution of twelve health centers across the nation. He is a visionary who, in his work as parish pastor, hospital chaplain, and professor of religion and medicine, sensed a need for a practical integration of religion and medicine. This conviction gave brith to his model of church-based health centers. The centers in affiliation with WHC, Inc. employ a physician, nurse and pastoral counselor in the health team. Centers in low-income areas often include a social worker.

Westberg opened the first holistic health center more than ten years ago in a Lutheran church in a low-income area of Springfield, Ohio. The next center opened in Hinsdale, Illinois, an affluent suburb of Chicago. The success of both convinced Westberg of the viability of his model for people in all income brackets. During the past two years Westberg and his staff in the national office have been experimenting with placing the model in settings other than a local church, such as within a home for the elderly and on a college campus.

Westberg has secured major support from a colleague, the director of preventive medicine at the University of Illinois Medical School. Major financial backing has come from the Kellogg Foundation, a large percentage of which has been designated for the opening of further centers throughout the country.

All centers affiliated with Wholistic Health Centers, Inc. utilize the health team. The presence of a pastoral counselor on the team insures that a person's relationship with God (or the absence of one) will be explored to the extent that it seems to have bearing on his or her total health. Each new patient completes a questionnaire related to basic life stresses and resources for dealing with them. This form is used in the health planning conference with the client and health team to help in assessing the person's total health, rather than focusing exclusively on the symptoms which have brought the client in for treatment. Doctors estimate that as many as 80% of the clients they see have used their present symptoms as an opportunity to share problems related to family, vocation or spirituality. The health planning conference provides a place for the client to share all his or her concerns and to participate with the health team in seeking a resolution for them.

Wholistic Health Centers, Inc. has been gathering statistics on both the cost effectiveness and the medical effectiveness of its model. Client testimonies suggest that whole person care is meeting a strongly felt need within the community.

One unique feature of these centers is the unusual degree of access to the professional staff. For example, pastoral counselors make home visits in the same way social workers do, in order to assess a particular family's patterns of interaction which might be more visible in the home over the supper table than in the counselor's office. Potluck dinners are held with the professional staff and clients. Evening seminars are organized around topics which concern six or more clients, such as how to stop smoking, psychology of women, aging, fear of the dentist, stress management, marriage, divorce, recent death and the grief process, living with terminal illness, family planning, and religion and therapy.

Counselors at these holistic health centers have discovered that the majority of counseling issues deal with areas of meaning, particularly the faith issues of commitment and surrender. Such a quest for meaning was certainly a central part of Helene's story.

The experience of one holistic health center patient illustrates this discovery even further. A 64-year-old man came to the center complaining of insomnia, weight loss, and loss of appetitie. "As soon as I take a bite or two I feel full and can't eat any more," he told the physician, who examined him and found no sign of organic disease.

At the health planning conference with the team, he revealed that he had lost his wife nearly two years earlier and since that time he had lived alone and gradually with-drawn from all family and social relationships. He rarely saw his daughter and son-in-law, who lived not far away, but they had finally persuaded him to come to the center. Several times over the course of a few weeks he visited the counselor who encouraged him to talk about himself and his situation. He was treated with kindness and respect, but with directness and honesty.

Gradually, he came to understand what he was doing to himself. He stopped smoking and started to eat and sleep better, and to visit his daughter and her family again. Eventually he moved into an apartment with two other men and got involved in a community art project for the elderly. He had been challenged at just the right time. He had been stuck in the grief process, unwilling to return to life, and visiting the clinic gave him direction and got him moving again.

Holistic health care centers often work closely with pastors in treating their clients. Paul Salansky, pastor of First United Presbyterian Church in Downers Grove, Illinois started referring members of his congregation to the center there, first for medical needs and later for emotional problems he did not feel capable of han-dling.

One of the primary reasons he refers people to the cen-ter is that he feels comfortable contacting the doctor, nurse, or pastoral counselor by phone or personally to ask if his own diagnosis was correct. They tell him the nature of the problem and indicate ways that he as a pastor can help that person, and how they can work together with the center if the person needs more treatment. This puts the church and the medical profession in a united relation-ship.

As Pastor Salansky says:

I see the Wholistic Health Centers as a tremendous asset to pastors. It lessens the fragmentation that occurs trying to figure out where to send people. I used to wind up sending a person to a physician in case a related physiological problem might be causing an emotional disturbance. The physician might send the person to a psychiatrist and from there, who knows where? That is not wholistic health. The team approach reduced the fragmentation.

A unique aspect of the personal health inventory utilized by WHC, Inc., clinics is the emphasis on one's own resources for getting well. Questions relate to goals, strong points and special abilities which will enable the client to reach the goals he or she establishes; also included is a chance for the client to assess his or her own physical symptoms and feelings, and to evaluate the help necessary to reach his or her goal.

The emphasis on stress-related illness and stress management may or may not survive its current popularity. Questionnaires about personal disease and stress history are not new. However, putting emphasis on the client's own resources for health and wholeness is unique. In contrast to the commonly held "fix-me" or "doctor-as-God" attitudes which perpetuates dependency, holistic care focuses on the possibility of recovery, even self-cure, based on inner resources on the path to wellness.

Several new holistic health centers are in the planning stages. Most of the existing centers are located in Illinois, including Chicago and the surrounding suburbs: Hinsdale, Woodridge, Oak Park, Oak Lawn, La Grange, and Mendota, Illinois. Two centers operate in Washington, D.C., as well as a center in Minneapolis.

This unique model of health care first occured to Westberg during his work as a hospital chaplain in 1944. He began to notice a correlation between hospitalization and recent loss. After running a small pilot questionnaire he discovered that more than ⅓ of all patients participating in the study could easily identify a loss that was responsible for a considerable amount of unresolved grief. Westberg verified his suspicion within medical circles, where he was told that at least 50% of patients seeing doctors are really dealing with grief related to interpersonal issues.

From these findings, Westberg developed a study on grief and health in which he outlined ten stages of grief which must be processed before a person is ready to move on to the next life challenge. He called this study *Good Grief,* and it remains foundational to all his later work in the area of whole-person care.

Westberg believes that illness related to stress, loss, grief, and life-changes usually comes on slowly. In other words, if the medical and helping professionals could put more emphasis on preventing illness, they might help people avoid a great deal of distress. Westberg points out that most *doctors* are trained to take care of crises—acute care situations—when in fact, most *people* fall into the category of being only mildly sick or disabled. Thus he made a two-fold appeal in his model of whole-person care: that more physicians should specialize in family practice medicine and treat the spectrum of general diseases rather than limiting themselves to an obscure specialization: and that physicians should not practice in isolation, but should utilize a team approach including a nurse and a pastoral counselor to help the client, since medical treatment is usually not the only issue present.

Westberg put his theories into practice during his time as professor of practical theology in Springfield, Illinois.

He established the Hinsdale center, which also houses offices for his national organization. Westberg summarizes his model of church-related health care:

> We have all these churches sitting vacant part of the week. They are easily convertible into a medical clinic weekdays and into Sunday school rooms on Sunday. The only exception is two small examining rooms which must be kept locked because of the equipment stored in them.
>
> The host church congregation is a participant in the healing process as it donates the space, heat, light, janitorial service, phone service and volunteers for the clinic's use.
>
> The Wholistic health care centers are not-for-profit corporations. Physicians earn about 75 per cent of a standard physician's salary, but clergy and nurses make an average wage.
>
> Clinics in churches can become self-supporting in about two years. Donated space and volunteers from the church help here, as do contributions from the community.
>
> To set up a wholistic health center in a community requires the approval of the county medical society, staffs of local hospitals, the local nursing society and the local clergy association.

Wholistic Health Centers, Inc. has experienced positive results in delivering health care in the church setting. Churches are usually located where people live and can often provide space within their buildings. The church setting is appropriate because of its long history of providing social services in the community. Church structures, in addition, symbolize the human spirit and its search for wholeness, a reminder that God is the source of healing. Church members often become dedicated volunteers ea-

ger to participate in providing whole-person health care,
belief in the close ties between medicine and religion. Ministers, according to WHC, Inc. are most often involved in
early cries for help and may have more innate skills than
they realize in dealing with the major causes of illness.

Westberg has officially retired, but his vision for health
care across the United States endures. His organization
has brought renewal to the American Health delivery system—providing creative models, teaching and encouraging care that revolves around the whole person, including
a role for the church in providing that care.

4 | What Are Its Theological Roots?

What do we really mean by "health"? What does "whole-ness" mean for service which is based on the Gospel? To what extent can the church, a congregation, promote whole-ness in its own individual members as well as in the commu-nity as such? What is meant by the "church's healing ministry"?

Contact, *Christian Medical Commission, WCC*

Jesus healed. He touched lame legs and gave them strength. He reached his hand to blind eyes and gave sight. He touched weak minds and restored order. He forgave sins and cast out demons, setting people free from spiritual, emotional, and physical bondage. After Pentecost, his disciples performed the same work of holistic ministry. The scripture clearly indicates that the church has been endowed with specific healing power. The reader of the gospels can readily perceive that Jesus invested a major portion of his ministry in healing the sick. Often, however, we have examined the individual healing miracles of Jesus, without considering the theological meaning of Jesus' healing miracles and the ongoing significance of those acts in the church's life today.

51

Healing and Wholeness

In considering the healing miracles of Jesus and the profound emphasis he placed on wholeness, we must ask
what Jesus wished to communicate through his healing
works in people's lives. That is best answered in the context of more basic assumptions about the meaning of
Jesus' overall ministry in and to the world.

Jesus was sent from God to usher in a new order of
creation, restoring the wholeness which God originally
bestowed upon the creation but which was shattered by
the fall. The resulting chaos and confusion is our partial lot
until the end-time; but God sent Jesus to begin a new
order in our midst. *Shalom* is the biblical word—and a
potent symbol—for the personal and corporate wholeness
in God's original creation. Through the power of Christ's
death and resurrection true wholeness can be recreated
out of the chaos which reigns on this earth. Old Testament
insights into the threat of reigning chaos and God's prom-
ise of *shalom*, expressed powerfully in the servant songs of
Isaiah as well as elsewhere, find their continuity and fulfillment in the life and ministry of Jesus (see Isaiah
65:17–25).

The healing miracles of Jesus, then, can be understood
as some of the first signs of the new order Christ pro-
claimed and inaugurated. These miracles are inextricably
bound up with the concept of the Kingdom of God, and
can best be interpreted as the first fruits of the new Kingdom. Jesus' healings are signs of the breaking in of the
Kingdom of God, in all its power, and point to the coming
time when the new Kingdom will be totally fulfilled.

This interpretation of the healing miracles of Jesus is
well presented in the provocative and valuable study,

Community, Church and Healing by R. A. Lambourne. Lambourne describes the healing work of Jesus:

> In the mission and message of Jesus Christ his healing work was not a secondary consequence, but the very means of proclamation, institution, and enlargement of the new age, the rule of God. . . . The healing works of Jesus are visible signs of the breaking through of the power of God, the Kingdom, the day of the Lord, and therefore they are both moments of salvation and judgement for the community in which the healing work is done.

Lambourne further describes the inter-relationship between the healing miracles of Jesus and the coming Kingdom of God as follows:

> When Jesus confronts men and women with powerful acts of healing he does not ask for mere wonder and awe; what he asks for is that men and women will recognize in the healing act a *theophany*, God's presence, his word, his finger. The response demanded of God's people when he appears is that they should repent and enter into the promises of the covenant.

The theological significance of the healings performed by Jesus Christ is that they witness to God's intention to restore wholeness for all people and all creation. They come to the hearer of the gospel as signs which underscore the meaning of the Kingdom which Jesus announces. To the follower of Christ, his healings testify to the spiritual power upon which that Kingdom is built, and upon which believers base their lives.

Christ gave the gift of healing to the church as a source of power, to act as a channel through which God's healing may flow. Faith and healing are integrally related as demonstrated in all the healings recorded in scripture. However, faith itself is a gift of God and cannot be produced by an act of will. It is not a quantity to be measured but a gift to be sought through prayer. Faith is part of the healing process, whether it springs from the heart of the one seeking healing or the person or community interceding for him or her.

Some involved in ministries of healing believe that there is a particular power in corporate prayer for healing. Scripture gives certain precedents for this view, particularly in James 5 where it speaks of gathering the elders for anointing, the laying on of hands, and prayer. When healings occur they are profoundly uplifting to the whole life of the church because of their graphic and immediate evidence of God's love, grace, and power among believers. Since healing is a gift given to the whole church, any individual can begin to appropriate this gift on behalf of another. Frequently, we do not have because we do not ask.

In the New Testament healing flowed from the fellowship of those who gave themselves to each other as Christ's body, the church. Charismatic theologians such as Morton Kelsey and Francis McNutt state that healing was a primary ministry of Jesus and his church, which fell into disrepute sometime during the Middle Ages, when the sacrament of anointing the sick became merely a rite for the dying. Kelsey, an Episcopal rector, researched his study of healing for fifteen years. He believes Christians must return healing ministries to the ordinary life of a congregation and de-mystify the experience of being healed by God of one's infirmities, whether they are emotional or physical, congenital or accidental.

If the church is to reclaim its healing ministry, it must ask the question, "what constitutes wholeness?" Wholeness is a dynamic process of working toward integration, toward harmony with oneself, with others and with the Creator. It is possible to know wholeness in the midst of a terminal illness such as cancer if one has reached a place of honesty and humility about oneself, a place of confession and forgiveness and the receiving of forgiveness. Wholeness does not simply mean a lack of physical or emotional symptoms. Although we strive for healing of troublesome symptoms, that manifestation of healing only occurs as a gift of God.

John Sanford, Episcopal priest and Jungian analyst, has written the provocative study *Healing and Wholeness.* Basing his arguments on the thinking of Carl Jung, he suggests that the cultural definition of health as adjustment and adaptation to cultural norms is false and needs revision. He reminds the reader that the whole society was sick in Nazi Germany, so that those who could not adjust or adapt to Hitler's views were not sick, but profoundly well. Sanford believes that life is a journey toward wholeness, but that wholeness is not the same thing as peace of mind. For Sanford, suffering is a necessary part of daily living and the process of becoming whole.

Suffering is a part of living. It always has the potential for transformation if, like Job and Paul, we are able to preserve our faith in the midst of it. No one is immune from suffering; on the contrary, the Scripture demonstrates that suffering serves a purpose in the lives of individuals. Sooner or later we have to examine the question of suffering, for it is painfully obvious that all who seek healing are not healed.

Healing and suffering bring us to the basic question of God's will. Although God's will remains the ultimate mystery, there are some aspects of it that are clear. God's will is dynamic, not static. God's will always calls the Christian to greater faith and hope. Regardless of the outcome of individual suffering, our primary calling is to be drawn into deeper relationship to God.

Ultimately, there should be no conflict. One can find resolution in the acceptance of this paradox: suffering exists side by side with supernatural healing. The faith and hope to pray for divine healing is not opposed to the faith and hope to accept what is given. But in both appeals we must always seek the transforming power of God's love.

Suffering is part of living. There is no escape. The only choice is whether we want to keep on saying "yes" or "no" to our lives as they are given, as they unfold. If we say "yes" to life, including suffering and death, there is potential for transformation of ourselves, and sometimes even our circumstances. We can learn to use whatever faith we may have to say "yes" to life and death. This choice is profoundly important because whether we are saying "yes" or "no" to life has more to do with our health than most other factors. True wholeness means being able to receive our circumstances and move on in faith.

The subject of suffering is relevant to us all; two books on suffering that are particularly useful are Rabbi Harold Kushner's book *When Bad Things Happen to Good People* and Philip Yancey's *Where is God When it Hurts*. Rabbi Kushner's book reflects the Old Testament truth of the unity of body, mind and spirit. Suffering belongs to us all whether Christian or Jew.

Confession and Healing in the Church's Life

People are not meant to embark on a journey toward wholeness alone. That is the basis of the Gospel. The fellowship of believers exists so that we can move together toward healing and reconciliation.

Psychologist O. H. Mowrer understands early Christianity as a small group movement. Individuals confessed and made amends within their congregations. Christianity spread, he believes, because this practice was so redemptive and rehabilitative. Mowrer thinks people should return to living in community, fully under the judgment and forgiveness of one's family and friends. In this context, religion could function literally as reconnection, reunion and reconciliation.

In an article on Integrity Therapy in the September, 1977 issue of *Faith at Work* magazine, Mowrer expresses a need for people to begin living up to their consciences. Honesty, openness, restitution and willingness to help others are basic to Mowrer's therapy. He defines openness as letting others see us as we really are—taking the injunction literally in James 5: "Confess your faults to one another."

In *Life Together*, Dietrich Bonhoeffer wrote:

> In confession, the break-through to community takes place, [Sin] withdraws [us] from the community. . . . Sin wants to remain unknown. It shuns the light. In the darkness of the unexpressed it poisons the whole being of a person. This can happen even in the midst of a pious community. In confession the light of the Gospel breaks into the darkness and seclusion of the heart. . . . It is a hard struggle until sin is openly admitted. But God breaks gates of brass and bars of iron.

Personal transparency and sincerity within our daily lives can lead to freedom from the nagging fear of being exposed for who we really are. In the process we can expect growing energy and greater health. It is a hard struggle to confess to one another, Bonhoeffer says, but those who have tried it believe this approach is a certain path to wholeness.

A further implication of healing in the church's life lies in the role of individual lay people. Healing is not the territory of experts; people of faith are asking how they can become healing agents for God. Some are particularly called and equipped for a healing ministry, but every Christian can act as a healer in his or her own life, and in those lives around him or her. Morton Kelsey and Francis McNutt offer some practical suggestions for appropriating healing in our daily living: 1) sharing a call to a particular healing work with others, 2) seeking to know God personally, 3) praying for our own healing and that of others, and 4) offering ourselves to others for their healing. This parallels the Alcoholic Anonymous recovery program—finding freedom in sharing one's confession of weakness and serving others still in bondage to their particular addiction.

In our enthusiasm for healing prayer, a word of caution seems wise. Since Jesus is the Savior and Healer, we must always seek his will as we consider praying for healing. Our primary task is to listen for God and to identify where, how, and *if* God may want to use us as we pray.

Whole-person health care is, therefore, the heritage of the church. We must reclaim our function as the primary mediator of healing in society. This is not an easy task. In order to become a healing church we must grant deeper and deeper access to one another. It will be necessary to sustain each other in this difficult process as we often battle against feelings of self-protective fear and revulsion. We must help one another to accept the brokenness we find in ourselves and each other so that we can engage in these much needed healing tasks.

What will it take to turn our local congregations into caring, healing communities where we are known one to another? We must pay a price for this style of living, just as in the intimacy of our family setting, we are often subject to hurt and disappointment. But if we fail to risk this intimacy with one another we are settling for an impoverished church. Releasing the potential for health and wholeness available through the message and experience of Christ's healing love may seem to be a risky venture, but the alternative is to spend our lives locked in to lifeless churches which do not choose to experiment with Christ's challenge to become a new family through his power. We will put in our time in weekly attendance, but will never be able to integrate our spiritual dimensions with our life in the world. We will not experience God's *shalom*, that experience of wholeness which results when we are living reconciling lives, available through the power of God's gathered community the church.

If it seems presumptuous or audacious to ask God for healing of ourselves and of the nations, we can remember that we are not responsible for the outcome. Not only is it possible, but it is our duty to pray with open hands, ready to receive whatever comes in hope and confidence in God's care for the world and for us.

Several years ago some dear friends gave birth to a child with Downs syndrome. Their response to this crisis provoked many of their Christian friends. They asked God to heal their child outright. This was the deepest cry of their hearts to a caring God. Through the years they have continued in their request. Although many have told them that there is a reason God allowed this sorrow to come their way and that they must not question God's wisdom, they have persevered in the belief that they can always ask their loving God to heal. They have been faithful in training their child to his fullest potential, while they wait in hope for indications of healing in whatever form they may appear.

I suspect that they were not wrong. I believe, in fact, that they have been profoundly obedient to preserve hope in God's intervention. Their whole family has experienced more wholeness in the midst of suffering and disappointment than those whose instruction was to "tough it out" in a manner more like stoicism than like Christian faith and hope. As Saint Paul wrote, "for now we see through a glass darkly, but then face to face. . . ."

What keeps us from experiencing more of God's healing touch in our churches? Fear of disappointment seems much to blame. It is a great freedom to sense that healing, like faith, comes as a gift. We can ask for it, we should do everything we can to promote wholeness in our lives and in the world around us, but in the final analysis we wait in hope for a gift. If we have the courage to live in this expectant hope of God's healing, the church can step forward in the power given in Christ to mediate this healing in our broken world.

One remaining question in this discussion of faith and healing is the relationship of medical science to divine healing. Many have difficulty synthesizing the "wonder drugs" of modern health care with the scriptural injunction of laying-on-of hands and prayer. Healing comes through physicians' hands as well as through prayer. These are not opposing forces to be pitted against each other, but the fullest utilization of both the rational and the intuitive aspects of humanity. Problems occur when we isolate and compartmentalize either source of healing. A wholly scientific approach lacks the resource of God's power, and a wholly spiritual approach overlooks God's confidence in human beings. The Divine Physician has authority over every tissue in our bodies. We must realize that all our illnesses are within reach of God's touch regardless of the medical, spiritual or emotional treatment plan we follow.

Maturity is marked by acceptance of God's sovereignty. Our will to experience healing may not reflect God's ultimate purpose for our lives. Yet we can find fulfillment while living amid the tension of God's yearning with us for wholeness, knowing that the deck is not stacked. We accept the fact that our lives include suffering and circumstances from which we will not always be healed. Caught between these two realities we can still pray in faith for God's healing touch.

Finally, becoming whole should never become a substitute for salvation, or a weapon with which we beat friends and family into an even deeper sense of guilt and failure when they do not respond to traditional medical treatment. It is painful enough to be sick, and even more painful if others imply that the one who is ill is not doing all he can to get at the roots of his sickness.

Yet in the midst of all these complex factors, wholeness in Christ is within our reach. Growth in Christlikeness and the love of God are the ultimate purposes of our lives. Being made physically, emotionally, and spiritually whole is a lesser goal, not the main reason for being. As the Westminster Catechism states: We exist to "glorify God and to enjoy Him forever."

Our lives are a journey toward wholeness, wholeness not to be experienced completely this side of paradise. *God* is the journey, and the journey's end.

5 | Where Is It Practiced?

At different times and in different places, a search for a healing theology and an effort to carry out a healing ministry has fallen to the churches when the evidence of unmet health needs has become so overwhelming as to make it impossible to ignore it a moment longer.

Miriam Reidy, Contact, *Magazine of the World Council of Church's Christian Medical Commission*

In the fall of 1977 I had just finished a chaplain internship at Children's Hospital in Washington, D.C., prior to graduating from Wesley Seminary with a degree in pastoral psychology. Then, I was introduced to Janelle Goetcheus, a medical doctor, in the living room of Elizabeth O'Connor's home, and what followed was an extraordinary example of God's guiding and leading in the lines of his people.

Both Janelle and I had harbored dreams for establishing a health center that would treat persons as a whole, a unity of body and spirit. Each of us, from our different backgrounds in medicine and pastoral counseling, had seen that health is inextricably bound up with personal feelings. We also had envisioned a clinic that would serve the needs of the economically oppressed. And, we each had had contact with Granger Westberg. So, we began to talk with Granger and his staff about beginning a holistic health center in the city of Washington—a center that would be rooted in the life of a local church.

In the spring of 1978 we prepared a proposal and shared our strong sense of calling with the Church of the Saviour and with Sojourners Fellowship. Through prayer and conversation, Mary Hitchcock, pastor in the Potter's House Church, agreed to serve as president of the board of directors, giving leadership to bring the health center into being. A space was located on Columbia Road and more staff were appointed. At the same time Janelle issued a call for a mission group to give primary support to the health center. The staff was drawn together in the same amazing manner.

A History of the Columbia Road Health Services

The story of Columbia Road Health Services begins with the articulation of a vision. We were called to respond to the need for a holistic health care center in the heart of Washington, D.C., a city clearly divided between rich and poor, black and white. A clear element of our call was to find ways to make the clinic one which would serve the needs of the poor of the inner city. We ourselves were not poor, yet we sensed a call to simplify our lives, and we grappled with the meaning of indentification with the poor.

Our health center did not come into existence to serve the rich of Washington, for we knew that they had the means to choose any medical and psychological care they desired, yet, we knew we would not turn hurting people away, rich or poor. In the midst of the wilderness of inner city health care, we desired to be a prophetic voice and a model of hope challenging the existing structures to examine their relationship to those they serve.

A second aspect of our call was to embody a broad ecumenicity. We enlisted the cooperation of the Church of the Saviour and Sojourners Fellowship. In time, we expected that our staff would include other faith communities, as it did. We sought to be open to those who shared a common calling to holistic health care which was rooted in Jesus Christ and in Christian community.

Those who responded to the call to build a holistic health care center formed a family which shared each other's journeys as persons struggling to become God's people. To some extent the health family was seen as a microcosm of community and church, although pastoring continued to take place in our respective churches. We sought mutually acceptable ways to grow together as Christians, such as corporate worship, prayer and scripture reading. In this way we were seeking to establish a quiet center which would sustain us and all who would come to participate in the center's life.

In order to fully realize our ecumenicity, we invited people from the Church of the Saviour and Sojourners Fellowship to become board members of the holistic health care center. The board and staff joined together to form the broader health family. Together we nurtured the vision and life of Columbia Road Health Services, and used our resources and experience to seek financial backing, a space in which to locate, equipment, and introduction to the health community in the District of Columbia.

We held one another accountable to the original vision. Eventually, new mission groups were established within the Church of the Saviour, who felt called to serve various aspects of the center's life. These groups searched out ways to involve others in offering their services and gifts. In this way Columbia Road Health Services was the realization of a dream and calling of many people whom the Lord brought together in service.

The elements of vision for this holistic health center were three-fold: to serve the poor, to be ecumenically staffed, and to form a faith community within the staff.

Another component of the vision was to build bridges between rich and poor within the city and the church. To that end fees were charged according to a person's ability to pay, and no one was turned away.

Columbia Road Health Services is a non-profit, tax-exempt and local church-supported physicians' family practice, with pastoral counseling and social work services. Each of us who constituted the staff and board members responded to a basic vision to provide health care which ministers to body, mind and spirit and to make that health care affordable. We strongly believed in and acted on "the right to health care."

In inner city Washington, D.C., located in an ethnic neighborhood composed of one-third black, one-third white, and one-third Hispanic population, we were overwhelmed by the needs of the poor among us. We charged for our services according to a person's income level and the number of dependents supported, but sometimes our clients could pay nothing for services received. Because of this, there was a constant need for contributions to offset the costs of providing care where it was required.

In order to respond adequately to Hispanic clients we sought out a bi-lingual receptionist who assisted in the examining room with Spanish-speaking people.

Our ministry of whole-person health care offered family practice medicine, pastoral counseling, and social services through a health team which included a physician, a nurse practitioner, a pastoral counselor, and a social worker. We also cooperated with Medicaid, Medicare, and private insurance. We made no profit and our staff worked at sacrificial salary levels. We looked for people who would support our work either by patronizing us and paying our full fees, or by making tax-deductible contributions. In this way, we could serve more low-income people.

Each patient at Columbia Road Health Services would sit down with the health team and share about basic life stresses and conflicts, a health history and potential resources for getting better. This approach was welcomed by our patients because people are eager to be seen in all the complexity of their beings. Together with our patients we search for the key to unlock better health and an improved sense of well-being.

There is a wellspring of resources within each person which, if tapped, can lead the way toward wholeness of body, spirit and mind. The health center explains to the public that it offers everything that a family practice physician does, plus the services of a social worker and a pastoral counselor.

Pastoral counselors are a key part of the church-based health center's total person care. Their presence enables the staff to be uninhibited and unapologetic about faith perspectives, and the role of faith in the care that is offered. The presence of these counselors also allows the physician, social workers and nurse to serve primarily as practitioners, without having to bear the primary responsibility of witnessing, but still allowing them to express their faith in the appropriate context of health care.

One of the center's strengths is simply the time available for each client. The average client spends thirty minutes with either the physician or the nurse, and clients have a feeling of being unhurried, knowing that professionals are there to serve them and that they have the freedom to ask questions. They can take the time they need to express other things that are going on in their lives. This leads to a more complete and balanced understanding of who they are and of the pressures that are being brought to bear on their health. Judi Floyd, the nurse practitioner, says many clients appreciate the special warmth of the center and the time taken by the staff to explain and interpret each case.

Another of the center's strengths is that the staff does not deal with clients in isolation. Instead, problems are discussed by the staff in weekly case conferences so that all aspects of the client's needs are taken into consideration. At times staff meetings are cut back to give case conferences more time.

The center also realizes its limitations, however, and does not hesitate to refer its clients to specialists. Even then a follow-up is maintained as often as possible.

Our experience in working with inner city people convinced us on the viability of bringing an expression of the church into the market-place of humanity, and making its ministries accessible to all people regardless of race, creed, sex, or economic status.

The response to the center has been profound. People from across the country and in other parts of the world have written to share in what we were learning in our practice of whole person care and in our faith.

The entire staff now includes two doctors, a nurse practitioner, pastoral counselors, a social worker, a business manager, a receptionist, and nursing and medical interns. Included are Roman Catholics, Presbyterians, and Mennonites, as well as ecumenical fellowships such as Sojourn-

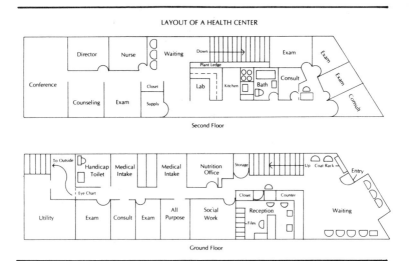

LAYOUT OF A HEALTH CENTER

Second Floor

Ground Floor

ers and Church of the Saviour. Two physicians, both of Providence Hospital, closed their laboratory and gave their equipment to the center. An enlarged center was dedicated to God's glory through the healing of the sick on December 20, 1981.

I served as Director of Columbia Road Health Services from 1978 through 1979. Our staff grew from three to ten in the first nine months. In each case there was a clear sense of each individual being called to our structure and to our life together. Three of the ten donated their services, including a nursing student, a member of our supporting mission group who was also a nursing assistant, and a gifted physician with a specialty in internal medicine and a burning desire to provide hospice care for the dying.

Although the vision has always seemed to exceed the financial resources, we have seen God's hand caring for us through money too. Our patient load has increased from a handful in the early weeks to over 10,000 medical, social work and therapy visits last year. Among our clients are many who have responded to our invitation to pay at the top of our sliding fee scale so that less fortunate others can secure care for little or nothing. The staff and board of directors have increasingly recognized the need to come together for prayer and reflection about its services and personal needs for wholeness.

Today, Columbia Road Health Center has been providing health care for poor people and others in the city of Washington for over three years. Our original location became so inadequate that the move to larger quarters became imperative for a more effective ministry.

The people who come to Columbia Road have taught us much. Paul is a sixty-nine-year-old gentleman who for twenty-eight years of his life had little health care. Ironically, during the months when his health reached a critical life-threatening point, he had many physicians, including specialists, involved in his care. His friend came several months after Paul became ill and asked us to visit Paul. Earlier, he had been released from D.C. General with a diagnosis of advanced tuberculosis; when he was released there were no arrangements made for him for food or income. When we saw him in his apartment he was very short of breath but refused to return to D.C. General.

Through pleading, we obtained emergency Medicaid and admitted him to Providence Hospital. Two days later he lay with no obtainable blood pressure and little other medical help for him. For the next four days Sister Marcella, our social worker, sat with Paul in the critical care unit. They talked about living and dying and about his negative experiences with white people.

He asked Sister Marcella to read the Bible to him; they prayed together, and Sister Marcella taught him to sing the Jesus prayer: "Jesus, Son of God have mercy." Paul would sing and add verses: "Jesus, Son of God, be with me, hold me, bring me peace, heal me," while the nurses in the critical care unit worked about him. Later in the week he was able to be moved back to a regular floor, and eventually back home.

As Sister Marcella spent time with Paul, she literally became Christ to him; thus we are to become Christ to each other.

A recent report from Columbia Road Health Services reveals their continued exposure to pressing needs:

> We are deeply aware of the suffering that takes place all around us. One of our patients is hospitalized, after suffering several strokes, and is not expected to live. One of our elderly patients, a double amputee, died in her bed as a result of a fire. Mr. William, a "bag" man living on Columbia Road has been coming in daily for treatment of an upper respiratory infection. He comes to us for a daily supply of his medicine, a cup of coffee, and confides, "I'm afraid I may freeze to death this winter."
>
> We are now seeing several persons who are living in half-way houses in the neighborhood with no place to spend their time or receive a little nurturing. A visit with the receptionist, the nurse, the volunteer, the physician, the social worker, and the promise that there will be another appointment next week, brings comfort and hope for the moment.

Dr. Goetcheus sees part of the answer to eliminating the barriers to quality health care for the urban poor in

. . . the establishment of primary care community centers around the city which would become centers of health care and social activities for the community. Dr. Goetcheus and the staff of the CRHS therefore see their own center as . . . a mini-model of what the larger system should be. It attempts to help persons see the integration of the physical, emotional and spiritual; to see themselves as whole persons.

A graduate of Ball State University in Muncie, Indiana and of Indiana University School of Medicine, Dr. Goetcheus spent three months serving in a Methodist Mission Hospital in Kapanga, Zaire in 1964–65. She is married, has three children, and is a member of the Church of the Saviour, Potter's House Faith Community. Her husband, the Rev. Allen Goetcheus, is a Methodist minister and director of Columbia Road Health Services. Dr. Goetcheus described the health needs of inner city Washington as follows:

The primary source of health care for the poor of Washington comes through the hospital clinic system—which is often dehumanizing, requiring 3–6 hour waits—a system in which the poor are maneuvered between multiple specialty clinics to see a different doctor each time they come, and with no one coordinating the health care. What happens is that many of the poor simply give up on health care rather than endure this dehumanizing care—and thus often develop serious illnesses that would never otherwise have developed. A reflection of this system is the infant mortality rate in Washington which is the highest in the nation—comparable to some Third World countries. One of our patients recently brought an underweight 7 month-old child to us. The mother had had no prenatal care, had gone to the hospital emergency room in labor, became discouraged waiting—left—came home and with the help of her elementary-school aged children delivered the baby herself.

Dr. John Karefa-Smart of the Howard University Hospital, Department of International Health who heard Janelle testify at a hearing regarding health care conditions in the District of Columbia, said: "Listening to these first-hand accounts of how little and how poor health care is available to the disadvantaged in the capital city of the world's most affluent nation was a sobering and maddening experience." These stories described the situation in Washington, D.C., but they are only an example of what is happening in a great number of other large Western European, North American or Austrialian cities.

The ministry of Columbia Road Health Services is grounded in responding to the cries of the poor. It is a ministry of hope to those it serves.

Vellore Christian Medical College and Hospital

Another model of whole-person health care is the Vellore Christian Medical College and Hospital in South India. There, an entire department is devoted to faith and healing. With strong Christian leadership, this hospital and medical college is striving to discover the meaning of whole-person health care, both in theory and practice. Vellore has the added dimension of rural health programs located in surrounding areas where health care exists in the context of nutritional, educational, and vocational programs directed toward the needs of the total person. The church in the West has much to learn from Vellore.

Eight out of ten people in India live in 560,000 rural villages. Yet, 80 percent of India's doctors are found in larger cities. Those in rural areas are afflicted with the most basic of health needs. One child in four dies before the age of four. With almost no sanitation, disease and infections run rampant. Malnutrition is a way of life for millions of these people, so the susceptibility to disease is intense. Pregnant women and infants are particularly vulnerable; inadequate nutrition invites disease which often can be fatal.

Innoculations or medicine against basic diseases frequently has not reached these areas, so malaria, tetanus, small-pox, measles, and other diseases which can be fully preventable, often become life-threatening.

One rural area not far from Vellore, India, called the K. V. Kuppam Block, is typical. Seventy-five percent of its 100,000 people fall below what the Indian government establishes as its poverty line, an income of about $95 per year. Only 32 percent are literate, despite intensive recent efforts of the government. About half the men have marginal reading skills, but only 12 percent of the women can read at all.

In its 45,000 acres there are eighty-three villages. Income comes almost exclusively from agriculture. For every 1,000 children born, 116 die at birth. Between ages one through four 23 percent die, mostly from diarrhea and dysentery. Forty-two percent of all deaths in the area are children below the age of five. Yet, the birth rate is 38 per 1,000, and the death rate is 29 per 1,000; the population, therefore, continues to grow, increasing the hardships of the people. This portrait of 100,000 people who live near Vellore is the story of modern India.

The needs of those who lived in the Vellore area of South India beckoned Dr. Ida Scudder at the turn of the century, over eighty years ago. Her one-room dispensary established in 1900 is now a 1200-bed hospital treating 27,000 in-patients and 392,000 out-patients each year who pay according to their means. The medical college begun from Dr. Scudder's ministry has now trained over 1400 doctors and 3100 nurses, and is regarded as perhaps the finest institution of medical learning in India.

Ida's father, Dr. John Scudder II, was a medical missionary following the path pioneered by his father, John, a member of the Franklin Street Reformed Church in New York City, who arrived in India as one of its first medical missionaries from the U.S. in the early nineteenth century.

Young Ida wanted no part of her family's legacy. One night, however, three different Indian men came to her family's home asking for her aid, for each of their wives was gravely ill. Knowing no medicine, Ida offered to get her father. The men refused his assistance, for customs both of Hindu caste and Moslem practice prevented a man from entering a home and medically treating a woman. Ida could do nothing. The next day she learned that all three women had died.

Ida believed she had heard God's call coming three times to her door. She went back to the U.S., entered medical school, and returned to India especially to treat women, beginning with the one-room dispensary in 1900. Thus began the Vellore Christian Medical College and Hospital.

Vellore's past is glorious, yet its present is largely unknown among many U.S. Christians who tell their children the story of Dr. Ida Scudder.

In a time when institutions have become increasingly secularized, Vellore remains focused clearly on its Christian identity and it demonstrates this identity through practice rather than mere rhetoric. Vellore treats the human person as a unity of body, mind and spirit. Its healing strives to be the healing of the whole person.

Rather than compartmentalized approaches that divide what is naturally unified, Vellore integrates the spiritual, emotional, and physical in its healing ministry.

Dr. L. B. M. Joseph, Vellore's Director, states, "In a Christian hospital, healing takes place in the context of worship and witness." Along with its medical excellence, Vellore's goals reflect the search to understand the meaning of pain, suffering, and death. In short, Vellore wants to bring the church into the heart of the medical world.

Involvement in the work and ministry of healing is not an optional calling, to be narrowly understood as applying to only certain believers. It lies squarely on the path of all who would follow our Lord. As Dr. Joseph states, "We are healed only to the extent to which we enter into the healing ministry of Christ."

From its earliest days, and in the vision and work of its founder, Dr. Ida Scudder, Vellore has lived out a Christian witness of focused compassion for those most afflicted, and most removed by reason of sex, caste, or economic circumstance, from the possibility of medical care. The institution has evolved in response to felt needs—such as its responsibilities within the emerging nation of India, and the commitment to become financially self-sufficient. From its evolution arose an understandable tension: to provide excellence in medical research and practice, developing the specialities of contemporary medicine, and serving all those who seek Vellore's outstanding care, yet to remain faithful to its original calling and mandate as a Christian institution, focusing its concern on the poor.

One of the presidents of the World Council of Churches, Cynthia Wedel, visited Vellore to attend a symposium on faith and health. After her return she commented:

The Vellore institutions are much more than a medical school and hospital. They stand out like a beacon of hope and help to a vast number of people who desperately need both.

In spite of severe over-crowding, and very limited facilities, the hospital is doing an amazing service. While they have able specialists and can give excellent and very sophisticated medical care, they seem to find a way to help the tragically poor who find their way to the hospital or one of its out-stations. The statistics on the percentage of graduates who go out to serve in the villages are impressive.

This unique institution, so rich in its history, is even richer in what it has to teach Western Christians about obeying Christ's command to heal. Ironically, an eighty-year-old mission hospital in the heart of South India stands on the cutting edge of the holistic health care movement, while health care in the United States is just beginning to integrate faith with medicine. The Vellore Hospital and College practices and teaches whole-person care, a reflection of the deep personal Christian commitment in the lives and work of many of its staff.

My initial contact with Vellore came at their consultation on faith and health, which prompted my first visit. At that consultation, I was surprised to find that the then Dean of the Religious Work Department, the Rev. A. C. Oommen, spoke with great depth of experience about the Christian Medical College and Hospital's attempts to bring the perspectives of Christian faith into the treatment plan of each patient. Concrete examples include a large chaplain's staff located at the heart of the physical plant, which receives each patient's chart and assigns a chaplain to each case along with the medical team.

The chaplains at Vellore are not superfluous, as they so often are in American hospitals. They are respected members of the health care team. Chaplains not only pray with the ill and dying patients; they sometimes make recommendations about how a particular illness may be a symptom of a deep underlying spiritual distress or crisis of faith.

According to Oommen, one of the primary goals of Vellore is to bring the church into the heart of the medical world. He believes that a major task of the chaplain's department is to turn every medical person into a chaplain. Rather than expressing the defensiveness that many Christian health professionals exhibit, Vellore takes the offensive in stressing the centrality of faith to health. Thus, the staff is concerned with bringing the message of Christ to the operating table. Christians are in the minority at Vellore, both in terms of staff and patients, but a core of leaders, committed to Christian vision and purpose, seeks to keep the hospital rooted in its heritage of Christian faith and practice.

Further, the chaplain's department concerns itself with making the Christian congregation an agent of healing. The chairperson of the Vellore CMC's council, Daisy Gopal Ratnam, reiterates this emphasis on the local congregation as a healing agent:

> The Christian concept of the healing ministry has gone through revolutionary changes from just being medical work in terms of meeting physical need, of providing avenues for the preaching of the Word, to the role of the local congregation in being the unit of faith and healing. The congregation is the primary agent of healing, and at the heart of this healing activity, lies the ministry of the Word, the Sacraments, and Prayer.

Vellore's approach to faith and healing rests on the conviction that healing means the restoration of a person to the purpose for which God created him or her. Healing involves much more than a cure. This broader definition of wholeness is part of our Biblical heritage, which shows us that healing miracles coexist with suffering from which there is no release. At Vellore, the staff has witnessed many "miraculous" healings, but it believes that any heavy emphasis on such cure hinders the opportunity for Christian growth and faithfulness in adversity.

The Christian Medical College complex also includes a mental health center where patients receive treatment in the company of a family member, so that the whole family can participate in both understanding the illness and providing the cure. Such family treatment is, in America, only in the beginning stages.

Vellore has also spawned a separate Christian counseling center which is international in scope, training pastors and lay people from churches in India and elsewhere to counsel those who are troubled. Students at the center participate as chaplains at Vellore hospital during their training program, an experience comparable to the training most American seminarians receive in hospitals as they prepare for ministry.

The Religious Work Department supports the medical staff as it grapples with the meaning of death all around. It attempts to build a supportive community to sustain its members as they battle with the fatigue which springs from the unceasing demands of the sick and poor of South India. The Religious Work Department ministers to patients, staff, and students. At present four assistant chaplains, two evangelists, and a librarian work with the Dean of the Religious Work Department. Daily services are conducted in English and Tamil, the language of the local province. Sunday worship is held in four languages, and Holy Communion is celebrated once a month in each language and given privately to patients in the wards by request.

During the past year the hospital has admitted forty times as many Hindus and Muslims as Christians, but chaplains visit the wards to offer counsel and a listening ear to every patient regardless of religious persuasion—and to pray with them, if they desire. The Department arranges training programs for counseling students from nearby seminaries and training institutions; it maintains, as well, libraries in the hospital and on the college campus. It offers retreats for spiritual growth, weekly Bible studies, and pastoral counseling. Further spiritual enrichment is enhanced by seminars on outstanding issues of the day, teaching missions with prominent speakers, work camps for the relief of disaster victims, and the publication of hymnbooks, prayerbooks, biographies, and addresses of notable Christians.

Another dimension of whole-person health care as it is practiced at Vellore is the emphasis on team treatment. Patients are treated by a physician, nurse, chaplain and occasionally a psychiatrist. Dr. L. B. M. Joseph, formerly a distinguished oncologist, characterizes whole-person care at Vellore:

> The ministry of healing whether it be in the city of New York, or in the continent of Africa, or at the Christian Medical College and Hospital, Vellore, or elsewhere in India is a part of God's plan for expressing His love and Christ's love to humanity, and for drawing humans closer to Himself, to remove discord, but more to re-establish that harmonious personality called the whole person.

Modern medical institutions are primarily concerned with the care of bodily ailments, with little regard or sensitivity to the whole personality and totality of life. At Vellore, as part of its care of the whole person, we have involved ourselves with the lives of neighboring communities in rural areas, not only in the field of preventive medicine and community medicine, but also in the field of total rural development such as agriculture, dairy farming, sericulture, adult education, child welfare, youth activities, nutrition, cottage industries, and family planning. Such a total involvement with the needs of the rural and urban community accepts the basic concept of health as harmony of the body with the environment, with society, and with nature and with God.

One such program called RUHSA (Rural Unit for Health and Social Affairs) directed by a committed Christian, Dr. Daleep Mukarji, has attracted international attention for the highly successful socio-economic development projects it is providing for the villagers within its specific target range.

RUHSA has recently received $150,000 dollars from the Ford Foundation to enhance the health and education of Indian women, for the potential of women in rural India has not been adequately understood. RUHSA will seek to influence the lives of many rural Indian families through strengthening the maternal and child care services available and through educating village women.

Another focus of attention at the Christian Medical College and Hospital has been the rehabilitation of leprosy patients. At Vellore the treatment of leprosy is an integral part of the hospital's medical responsibilities, and the study of leprosy is part of the academic responsibility of the teaching hospital. Two extraordinary specialists,

Cocherane and Brand, inspired their students and colleagues by example and precept, succeeding in getting them to touch leprosy patients without gloves and to treat them like any other patient. Their Christian witness was to remove the prejudice of leprosy from the minds of the doctors and the physician trainees, and to help the leprosy patient be accepted as part of their caring responsibility. A further testimony to their success is the New Life Center, a permanent residential leprosy rehabilitation center located on the medical college campus.

One of the newest forms of caring for the whole person at the Christian Medical College and Hospital is the center for mentally handicapped children also located on the college campus. Under the direction of a graduate of CMC, Sally Date, this center treats handicapped children in the company of a parent or relative over a three month period to help maximize the child's potential. Focusing on the strong Indian family ties, the center for handicapped children accepts any patient and family member willing to accept residential treatment and tries to show each family that their child is actually capable of more than is being expected in the home setting. Through a process of education and support for family members, the center seeks to teach the relatives to integrate their children into their family and village life.

The center accepts children with Downs syndrome and other chromosomal abnormalities, as well as those who have received injuries during birth or suffered other types of birth defects. Since many relatives cannot give an accurate history accounting for the child's disabilities the center concerns itself with potential rather than cause. They try to help families recognize that the treatment received at the center is the beginning of a lifelong process of training for their mentally handicapped child.

Many parents come hoping for a cure. They have come to believe that anything can be cured at Vellore. Often they have traveled great distances hoping for a miracle. Some are disappointed by the discovery that the treatment is a training program, not miraculous cure, and they leave. But those who stay are rewarded by new ways to relate to their children and hope for future improvement.

Psychiatrist Ambraham Verghese, Director of the Mental Health Center, finds that family support is very important in the treatment of psychiatric patients. He has been practicing family participation in mental health care for 25 years. He insists on the close relatives staying with mental patients in the hospital. They are provided family units so that each family can stay in the hospital independently. The relatives stay with the patients, being with them during treatment procedures, and giving them emotional support. Many psychiatric disturbances are caused by intrafamily conflicts, and these conflicts must be sorted out for the recovery of the disturbed patient. In most cases of psychiatric disturbances, the outcome of treatment is poor when there is no family support.

As Dr. Verghese says: "All of us involved in the treatment are joining hands with God to help the patient to come into fellowship with God, to help him to view his illness in the context of the purposes God has for him, thus it is essential that we in the healing profession have spiritual experience to draw on."

Dr. Verghese describes the relationship of faith to health in his experience as follows:

It is a fact that faith will enhance recovery. The placebo effect must be accepted. A faith that helps one to put his complete trust in God who is Love and who is all powerful, and a faith that will help one to accept the will of God in any situation, is a powerful force in healing. There is growing evidence to show that in conditions such as infections and even in cancer, the process of healing is faster when there is strong faith on the part of the patient.

This is even more relevant in psychiatric disorders. The relationship between the therapist and the patient is the most important aspect of psychotherapy, and the basis of this relationship is faith. This faith becomes all the more powerful if it is based on the omnipotence of God, the faith that gives the conviction to the patient that God is acting in the therapy situation, and that the person who is treating him is only a tool in the hands of God.

Faith gives courage to the person to live fully in this world, to take risk and to hope for the future. It removes despair and a sense of meaninglessness which are the cardinal features of neuroses and personality disorders. People get these psychiatric disturbances not only because of frustrations in life, but also because they are troubled about their destiny and the meaning of their existence. I believe that Christian faith helps one to get over these problems.

Perhaps one reason Vellore succeeds in its attempts to provide care for the whole person is its emphasis on remaining a vital Christian institution. It has never been preoccupied with defining holistic health care. Rather, from the beginning it sought to express the call of Christ to minister to the sick, the poor, and the outcast. In so doing, it has become one of the world's foremost examples of whole-person medicine in practice.

Clearly, wholeness at Vellore revolves around relationship to God. As Dr. Joseph put it, "Wholeness is harmony; disease is discord." Although Vellore has developed highly specialized care, it does not worship the advances of science and technology; nor has it lost its focus on the soul in the quest to master the diseases of the body.

The Scudder family and others came to India to communicate the Gospel in a land that little knew the message of Jesus. Now the Church of South India and the Hospital and College at Vellore have a message for Christian health professionals and church people of the western world. They witness to an understanding of wholeness that includes suffering, and they remind us of the basic role of faith in health and in the shaping of medical practice.

The Christian Medical College and Hospital is a testimony to vital Christian health ministries in the United States because it manages to incorporate the whole message of the gospel. It responds to the overwhelming needs of its people, the destitute of India, and it is not ashamed of striving to be Christian. While many American institutions still suffer from the compartmentalization of body and soul, of science and faith, Vellore has maintained what many western institutions have lost—unity of personal beliefs with professional practice.

The rapidly expanding holistic health care movement in both the church and the secular world indicates a growing sensitivity to this false separation. We are just beginning, but we have in the Vellore experience a wealth of wisdom and inspiration. If God is allowing us to do a new thing in health care today, Vellore can inspire us to be grounded in the basis for holistic health—Christian faith.

6 | How Can the Church Respond?

It is my conviction that the church's hour has come. The Church instituted by God, the servant of God, must again become his instrument to effect the synthesis for which all (men) of our time are consciously or unconsciously yearning. And here I mean the church in the broadest sense, not only the clergy, not only the established churches, but all those who have been gripped by Jesus Christ.

—Paul Tournier

Once we have gained a new sensitivity to those qualities which identify the church as the healing community it was created to be, we may wonder how we should respond. What appropriate steps can be taken to return healing ministries to the center of the Church's outreach? A local parish can create a health and healing ministry team in order to bring these concerns into focus in the church's life. However, many other options may be developed either alone or within a study group established to examine health and wholeness in the church's life.

One of the first tasks of any local church wishing to become involved in a health and healing ministry is to raise the consciousness of its membership in this area of

the church's ministry. In order to educate members effec-
tively, the pastor could preach a series of sermons on
Jesus' healing ministry followed by an overview of church
history, including reflection about why healing fell into
disrepute in the middle ages and how it is appropriate to
return these ministries to the ordinary life of the congregation, rather than confining healing to fringe groups outside the major focus of church concern. After this initial
introduction, a group could be formed to study health and
healing ministries in depth. There is a wealth of material
available on the subject (see Appendix). Another place to
begin is to assess the current areas of health ministry to
discover what already is serving the area of health and
wholeness in the church's life.

Some congregations may wish to establish a holistic
health care center using their facilities. Others may wish to
sponsor a center located in a more neutral building space
in the community. Sometimes existing Christian counseling centers and medical practices may wish to find a way
to cooperate through cross-referral or combining their services. There are almost endless possibilities for the creation of a health center. Some centers focus on the elderly,
some on the dying, and still others on the physically or
emotionally handicapped or on the poor. At Columbia
Road Health Services, Washington, D.C., there has been a
special focus on the Hispanic population including the
problems of illegal aliens seeking health care.

A local congregation starting a center must discover its
unique focus, not only to define a reason for being, but to
aid in fund-raising. Those considering funding such a project will be asking what distinguishes this project from the
hundreds of other bids for funding which they receive
daily. If your parish can identify a unique focus for minis-

try, it can be assured that its grant-writing efforts will be rewarded. Even in difficult economic times, the rich are as ever-present as the poor. Money is available. If a call is sensed and confirmed to begin this type of ministry, faithful commitment to bring it to fruition will be rewarded.

Another option is to begin a task force or interest group on whole-person health care within the congregation. At the very least, individuals can become more informed consumers when they visit the doctor. If the doctor does not make these vital connections the patient can. Who is in a better position to assess the whole of our lives than we ourselves? We need only take some time to find out about ourselves.

Every church will not be called or able to establish a health center. However, every congregation has the potential to establish its own health ministry team, which can greatly assist the pastors in meeting the health concerns of the parish.

A first step is to identify those members who are already involved professionally in health related fields. Additionally, there are many lay people with a keen interest in health needs who might wish to participate. A congregational health team may or may not evolve into a full health service; the main concern is to become a resource in the congregation for those with health problems. My own congregation has identified several areas of emphasis: medical skills, physical fitness, counseling, nutrition, prayer, and general help for the sick.

A congregational health team can establish its own limits. For example, those in the medical profession who have been assessed and screened by the pastors should be called on primarily for consultation and in emergencies. Obviously, there must be a clear understanding of how the health team is to be utilized, so that inappropriate expectations do not develop. The health team would not be a substitute for regular care from a physician or counselor. However, it might provide a meaningful supplement and provide a concrete way for a congregation to care for its members. Certainly it would be a first step to restore some aspects of the church's role in the healing process, a role which remains in need of repair.

The health and healing ministry team of Community Covenant Church, Missoula, Montana, has held seminars dealing with Christian approaches to whole-person health care, and produced a brochure which informs both members and visitors of the assistance available in the areas of counseling, nutrition, fitness, prayer for healing, and medical consultation. They have also established a prayer room which members may use at any time, but particularly in conjunction with the weekly communion service. Individuals may request prayer for healing of specific illness or interpersonal distress and may be anointed with oil, a common practice in the early church.

Some may object to the emphasis on the laity in establishing these ministries. However, church members often respond with more commitment when more is required of them. Apathy is more often related to being under-utilized than to being over-extended. Another concern for some may be the fact that many lay people do not have professional expertise and training in either the medical or helping professions. But it is a documentable fact that people respond to caring empathetic listening regardless of professional status. Many aspects of health and wholeness are directly related to feelings; a sensitive heart equips lay volunteers for such ministry.

At the Church of the Saviour, in Washington, D.C., small

Mission groups meet weekly for the purpose of Christian fellowship and discipleship in both the inward and outward journey, as their major spokesperson, Elizabeth O'Connor, has expressed it. Much inter-personal healing has taken place within these groups. The church is strongly committed to God's call outward in its mission to various aspects of the world's multiple needs, becoming instruments of healing in the lives of those they touch. The mission groups utilize disciplines of Scripture reading and meditation, prayer, tithing, corporate worship and a specific mission project. These groups provide a sense of family within the larger congregation and foster health and wholeness through a sense of belonging and a context for deeper fellowship and worship.

Many congregations have adapted the Church of the Saviour's model of small mission or *koinonia* groups for the purpose of individual accountability and nurture in the Christian pilgrimage. Often these groups aid in keeping people well because of the sense of meaning and purpose they fulfill as well as the primary support they provide. In a jet-age culture where most of us have lost connections with our extended families, groups like these can become our family, fulfilling a critical dimension of human existence.

Another congregation, Third Reformed Church in Holland, Michigan has utilized the Stephen ministers program, which trains the laity in pastoral care of those in the congregation who face life crises and severe stress. Those who have become Stephen ministers participated in a training program which equipped them to be helpful to members in crisis. The Stephen ministers assist their clergy in ministering to the needs within the congregation. Third Church has also offered an adult study seminar on

whole-person health care as a way to inform the membership of church-related health care and to determine what
type of involvement Third Church may wish to have.

The Voice of Calvary Ministries in Jackson, Mississippi,
founded by John Perkins, has been involved for 20 years
in black Christian community development through the
church, and both directly and indirectly in health care development. The Christian Community Health Fellowship
came into being as a result of VOCM's efforts in physician
recruitment and health care development.

H. P. Spees, who founded the Christian Community
Health Fellowship out of his work with Voice of Calvary,
had found a deep interest among Christian health professionals in the needs of the poor. Spree recalls:

> We sensed a real felt need and yet a frustration from many
> folks because of the lack of visible models for Christian
> community health care that at once reached the poor with-
> out paternalism and also was part of a larger, effective re-
> sponse to the need for community development.
>
> CCHF is a clearinghouse of ideas and opportunities
> where people interested in starting or supporting a Chris-
> tian health work in poor communities can write and get
> information.

Its objectives are to locate, recruit, and encourage Christian health professionals to use their skills in living out the
Gospel of Jesus Christ through health care in poor communities and to see Christian health projects become a
part or even the threshold to a comprehensive approach to
community development that meets people's spiritual,
physical, mental, emotional, and social needs.

The Christian Community Health Fellowship, in cooperation with other groups, have developed a preceptor-
ship program for medical students seeking exposure to

health care among the rural poor in Mississippi. The program includes study at the John Perkins International Study Center to learn basic strategies of Christian Community development.

On August 29, 1981, Voice of Calvary Family Health Center was dedicated in Jackson, Mississippi, the fourth health service affiliated with Voice of Calvary.

Medical and helping professionals and students in this training have a unique opportunity to develop effective black leadership in Mississippi through the resources of a nurturing interracial fellowship gathered at Voice of Calvary. Many Christian health professionals have had little exposure to the issues of racial reconciliation and justice or to the simple lifestyle of the rural poor. Yet these factors are as much a part of whole-person care as the more obvious spiritual links.

The Rev. Robert Baylor, Vice-President of Religion and Health, Evangelical Hospital Association, works with five greater Illinois hospital programs originally affiliated with the United Church of Christ. Within all five hospitals there has been a growing awareness of the validity of whole-person approaches to medical care, including acute care. Principles of holistic health care have been implemented throughout all levels of these hospitals, from nurses' training programs to primary patient care.

A woman in her 50's, a patient in Christ Hospital, recalls: "One of the important memories of my stay at the hospital is that the nurses and other employees were really concerned about me as a human being. They obviously cared about me as they cared for me, and that was a major factor in making my stay easier. I'm grateful for the spiritual climate that helped my recovery."

The Evangelical Hospital Association has employed Jill

Westberg, of Wholistic Health Centers, Inc., as a consultant in the area of holistic medical practice. They are on the forefront on church-related hospitals in the United States adapting holistic health care practices to the hospital setting. The EHA's programs include Christ Hospital, Good Samaritan Hospital, Good Shepherd Hospital, Bethany Hospital and Woodlawn Hospital. They also include Evangelical School of Nursing, a Wholistic Health Center in Oak Lawn, operated by Christ Hospital, and United Church Residences, rent-controlled housing for senior citizens and the handicapped.

Paul Umbeck, President of the Evangelical Hospital Association, summarizes their outreach as follows:

> The ecologist Dr. Barry Commoner has said there are three laws to ecology: 1) everything is connected to everything else; 2) everything has to go somewhere; and 3) there's no such thing as a free lunch.
>
> One of the prime lessons of the Evangelical Hospital Association's 75 years has been that everything is connected to everything else. Spiritual principles blended with loving human beings and superior technology created a healing climate that encourages wholeness—of the body, the mind, and the spirit.

A number of church-related hospitals are beginning to explore what their Christian heritage has to teach them in terms of caring for whole persons. Roman Catholic Hospitals such as Mercy in Muskegon, Michigan, and St. Patrick in Missoula, Montana, have made overtures toward implementing whole-person care within their programs. Deaconess Hospital of the United Church of Christ, St. Louis, Missouri, has the tradition of employing an ordained minister as chief executive officer in order to keep the concerns of the spirit present with medical care. Their president emeritus, Dr. Carl Rasche, visited the Christian Medical College and Hospital at Vellore to participate in the consultation on faith and health in February of 1980. Dr. Rasche reported that Deaconess was opening a laboratory to study psychosomatic illness.

Hospitals are beginning to compete for patients in these difficult economic times. Clients are in an excellent position to negotiate for whole-person approaches to their care, whether in giving birth or in the treatment of terminal illness, tonsillectomies or meningitis. As hospitals begin to succeed with whole-person care, others will follow.

The Lutheran Church has been very visible in whole-person health care. The Missouri Synod has a council for Christian Medical work, one of the few remaining medical desks in any major denomination. Their administrator, Florence Montz, R.N., is also involved in a pan-Lutheran organization devoted to health and healing, the Wheatridge Foundation which has done major research in the healing ministry of the church. Wheatridge sponsored a symposium on health and healing ministries of the Church in March, 1980, which is still influencing church-related health professionals. The major insight from the Wheatridge meeting is that the local parish is pivotal in the ministry to whole persons. Six parish-based models demonstrated new and creative ways for local churches to become involved in a health and healing ministry.

Wheatridge has prepared a Bible study on the healing ministry of Christ and continues to promote the role of the local church in the healing process. Robert Zimmer, President of the Wheatridge Foundation, describes his organization's purpose:

The Wheatridge Foundation observed a growing concern among congregations to find new and better ways to minister to the whole person. Models that provide ministries of mutual caring and compassion, of health and healing have been designed to "blend" with traditional programs of Word and Sacrament.

Minister and psychologist Donald Tubesing, one of Westberg's assistants in the early days of Wholistic Health Centers, Inc. has founded Whole Person Associates in Duluth, Minnesota. Both Tubesing and his wife Nancy are actively engaged in promoting whole-person health care through the publication of many books and tapes as well as workshop leadership and consulting with people and organizations desiring information and training in whole-person medical care. Tubesing's recent book, *Kicking Your Stress Habits*, makes valuable contributions to the study of stress-related illness.

The Reformed and Christian Reformed denominations sponsor the Christian Health Care Center in Wyckoff, New Jersey, a residential facility which attempts to provide Christian spirit with medical care for psychiatric and nursing home patients. This organization was founded by a group of Deacons of the Reformed, Christian Reformed and Netherlands Reformed churches and still receives major funding from these denominations.

Many ministries could be added to this brief survey. We are on the eve of an era of church responsiveness to the needs of whole persons. These varied examples of health and healing ministries within local churches and church organizations provide valuable insight and inspiration for other churches, serving as models for church-related holistic care.

7 | Marks of The Healing Church

Out of darkness shall come dawn;
Out of winter shall come spring;
Out of striving shall come peace;
But by the power of God.

—*Chinese Christian poet*

Addressing a large body of health professionals at the Shoreham Americana Hotel in April, 1978, Ruth Carter Stapleton, lecturer and author concerning inner healing, cited five root causes of illness: fear, frustration, guilt, insecurity, and loneliness stemming from rejection.

No one has escaped the experience of rejection, a fundamental experience of human life so painful that it often results in devastating consequences. Chief among these consequences is the lack of ability to trust, which the eminent psychologist Erik Erikson tells us is the foundation of the capacity for religious faith and belief.

Although there is little anyone can do to prevent an encounter with rejection, there is a role the church can play in the communication of God's acceptance of us as we are—a powerful balm for those smarting from rejection. And living our lives in the context of meaningful relation-

ships within our church life may have a direct connection
to our overall health—as it did for Helene.

The Needs of the Hurting Church

People cannot survive alone. Fellowship and a sense of
participation in the human community are essential to
health and well being. If we hate and judge ourselves
harshly, however, we cannot accept failure in others. Perhaps the more we can accept ourselves and our many
contradictions, the more we will be able to offer an uncon-
ditional acceptance to others. We are unable to be what we
have no models for in our own experience. If we are to be
God's ministers of reconciliation, we cannot afford to overlook Christ's messages of compassion and acceptance.

All of New Testament literature resounds with imagery
of light. Christ is the true light who has come into the
world to deliver us from darkness. But what kind of
darkness?

The darkness of sin takes many forms, but the most real
is an inner darkness, something akin to the "dark night of
the soul" so often referred to in mystical Christian literature and by poets whose imagination is captured by the
starkness of this image. In the poem "Desert Places,"
Robert Frost concludes his thoughts:

> They cannot scare me with their empty spaces
> Between stars—on stars where no human race is.
> I have it in me so much nearer *home*
> *To scare myself with my own desert places.*

Many of us can identify with Frost at this point. We live
with a vivid sense of our own desert places. And, in fact,
to some of us the Christian life can often seem to be a

continuous journey through the desert, whether we experience that desert within our own hearts or in our life circumstances. Life does not make sense. Things do not work out as we think they should. We struggle on, but we are discouraged and often overcome by these desert places.

What is the message of the Christian faith in the face of all of the desert places? In the *Advent of God*, Johannes Metz says that the malady of the contemporary person is the deliberate effort to forget the coming of God into human history, because that event, in its full impact, places a heavy demand on us. It demands that we relinquish the controls over our own life, accept change, and undergo complete transformation.

Metz continues, "Our faith tells us that God comes down to us. He is ever coming down to us and weaving Himself into *our historical Pageant*. We can never say that we have been born too late. We can never say that we missed God's coming, for our awesome encounter with Him still lies ahead of us."

The trouble is not that we have never experienced the coming of God into our lives. We have known that inbreaking of God into our lives and for a time lived on what seemed to be another level of existence. Life's circumstances seemed clear and real, and we felt as if we knew how to live because of the life we had discovered in Christ. But we forget, we cannot sustain the kind of faith relationship which enables us to transcend the ordinary and the petty—our everyday need to control everything and everybody around us. So we find ourselves back on the ash heap—back in the desert places, trying to avoid the memory of Christ, the coming of God into our lives which was so graphically real and enabled us to sense the meaning, if only for a brief moment, of losing ourselves in order to find ourselves.

The desert places have a hold over many of us. They do come back to encroach on that taste of freedom and to pull us back into hiding, back to low-risk relationships to God and to each other.

How do we guard against this kind of disheartenment—against the *malady of forgetfulness* as Metz names it? Or how, concretely, do we prepare ourselves to let God in?

Only with the aid and support of brothers and sisters in Christ, only in fellowship within our community are we drawn back to the heart of our call—the call to let God come and break into our existence with all the joy and the pain that such recognition and responsibility carries. The armor of light is love and reconciliation among us who call ourselves by God's name—something much easier to talk about than to live. To live a reconciled and loving life with my brother or sister demands of me that I be deeply rooted and grounded in the faith and trust that I belong to God and that that same relationship to God exists between each of my brothers and sisters.

On the countless occasions when I sense myself to be out of step with my brother or sister, when I am feeling hurt and angry and misunderstood, I must stand back and take stock. I must remind myself that God is also the God of my brother or sister. We have the same loyalty and vocation. Love bears all things, believes all things, hopes all things—and, we could add, dispels all things. For once we have established the real context for our human relationships, our common belief and relationship with Christ, the issue which was blocking our communication can be dispelled.

Either our Christian faith rekindles our waning hope or

it does not because we *cannot allow it to*. There is no satisfying explanation for all the desert places, places of struggle in life's journey except perhaps that Christ had them, too. But in the context of the Body of Christ I can be reminded and loved into opening myself once again to Christ's coming and all that that can bring into my life, if I am not too afraid to follow.

It is not our duty to succeed at being a healer. But it is our Christian responsibility to bring people into deeper dialogue with the faith dimension of their lives. Some may believe themselves agnostic or atheist, but particularly in facing death and loss, there is a very primitive kind of spiritual thinking that goes on within us all. Here the church can help us. Healing is available to people in the context of Christian community.

As wounded healers we discover that a mutuality exists between helper and patient. If I know myself to be hurt in certain areas, I do not feel removed from the patient. I know that I am a fellow pilgrim with those I meet; the most authentic questions we can raise with people are questions that come out of our own struggle.

Another thrust of the church's healing task is to enable people to see that God loves them as they are. In my home town and my church, as in Helene's, open sharing about failure was not encouraged. A person's struggle with alcohol or with a marital problem was interpreted as failure: Christians never got their hands dirty. Yet part of living is to sin, to make errors in judgment; when we live in Christ, these catastrophes can guide us into God's grace.

Part of the Christian calling is to share a God who is accessible to people. If people have rejected faith background because it was built on attaining perfection, they need to know that God accepts our humanity.

We need to learn to depend on the power that is mediated through the shared life of Christian community. In small support groups, in the larger community of worship and sharing, we can work together at building community. In small support groups, in the larger community of worship and sharing, we can work together at building community. In such fellowship we learn to face ourselves, to grow spiritually and emotionally.

Another source of renewal is the Eucharist. The experience of the Eucharist is especially meaningful for we learn to accept our own limitations and God's restoring love. When I come to worship I may be unreconciled in a number of relationships. If I took the scriptural injunction literally, I would not come to the table because I have not taken the steps of reconciliation. But I receive power to admit my sins and then begin to take action for reconciliation. Sometimes we have to live with our grievances until we receive the confidence or healing to go to a brother or sister and start working on our relationship.

In our church fellowship we try to accept the fact that each one of us has peculiarities and brokenness. Because we are broken people seeking wholeness, we try to stay in dialogue through the difficult times. Fleshing out this commitment is a very tension-fraught process, and relationships are often tried. Yet the victories deepen our fellowship in the midst of our mutual brokenness.

The Marks of the Healing Church

What characterizes the shape of the healing church—the church which is willing to act as a primary mediator of healing both to the wounded within its own membership and in society at large? The church has a rich healing potential, but the realities often fall devastatingly short. In fact, the church has often promoted sickness and sick religion rather than health and healing. This is particularly true when religion is used to express personality rigidities through religious devotion.

The question, then, becomes whether the ideal healing potential of the church can be made reality—whether the church can redefine its purpose and rediscover its humanity. A perpetual problem within the church is the existence of the "white sepulchures" which Christ rebuked. Ironically, fellow sinners within the church's life labor arduously to project the shadow which clouds their own lives onto the "other"—the "other" race, class, sex or economic groups.

We must be honest with one another. The church, if true to a Biblical understanding of itself, knows that *it* is the sinner and the outcast—ultimately unworthy of the grace extended to it through God in Christ. Throughout salvation history, the people of God have gone the way of the harlot for whom Hosea mourned and lamented. When we lose perspective on our true identity as the people of God, we cut off the possibility of becoming the healing body we were instituted to be. When we in the church have learned to accept who we are—the broken people Christ came to restore—we can extend the compassion of Christ in an authentic way.

There are a multitude of churches, yet so few healed individuals. Most of us in the church have resisted casting our lot with the emotionally poor and oppressed, just as we have failed to recognize and respond to the literal poor and their minimum survival needs. Dorothee Soelle suggests in her book *Suffering* that only those who themselves suffer can recognize and respond to the suffering of those around them. We must make friends with the pain within ourselves in order to transcend it and move toward overcoming the fear and loathing we instinctively feel for those who blatantly exhibit their poverty either emotionally or economically. Making friends with pain does not suggest resting there, but it may be a beginning place for those of us who instinctively turn from what is painful and repugnant in ourselves—and in our brothers and sisters.

One of the primary messages for the church today is that we who are the poor, we who are in sin, are called to serve the poor as healers of the whole person—emotionally, spiritually, and economically, for the total reshaping of our lives as God's people. We in the church cannot be a healing church until we know who we are—the people who have walked in darkness and have seen a great light. And if we are a people called by God to be that light which we have seen and experienced, then we must determine what it is that makes a church a healing church.

The first mark of the healing church is that it must be *home*—the home, in the ultimate spiritual sense, for which most of us have been seeking all our lives. The church must be a home which is only available to the undeserving. Robert Frost's powerful poem, "The Death of the Hired Man" describes such a home:

> Home is the place where, when you have to go there,
> They have to take you in.
>
> I should have called it
> Something you somehow haven't to deserve.

Frost has captured the paradoxical nature of the home that the church must always strive to be: a "place where when you go there they have to take you in," and at the same time, a place you somehow "haven't to deserve."

The church is called to be the kind of place where people have to be taken in, embraced, received in all their human misery and creative potential in order to be healed. This model of the servant church is reflected in the servant songs of Isaiah, and was carried out in the life and ministry of Christ Jesus. If we are interested in being faithful, we must re-evaluate ourselves in terms of the servant posture of Isaiah and of our Lord. What does it mean to be willing to be a servant people? Certainly for the church it means taking in whomever is sent.

Beyond simply opening the door to someone whom we would not choose, we are to create an atmosphere of caring. There must be a climate of love in which individuals are set free to tell their story and to find, at last, a resting place. Individuals in the church may not necessarily have unusual gifts of insight or healing; with or without such gifts, the church was intended to be a resting place, a home for our whole beings, the place where we explore ourselves in the context of salvation history. The church was designed to embody the "home for the heart" that Bruno Bettleheim and others have had to create outside its boundaries because they could not find it in the church.

Another mark of the healing church is that it is to be a *new family*. The concept of the "new family" in Christ is as old as the inquiry of Jesus, "Who is my mother and my brother?" The cost of becoming family in the Biblical sense is so high that most of us in the church have chosen the path of least resistence. We choose what is familiar. The nuclear family is a product of recent history, particularly within American culture, but it is not the picture of family given to us in Scripture.

In the church today, we tend to accept the predominant

understanding of our culture, the nuclear family, which is often the least demanding, yet the most fragile setting for enduring human relationships of caring and love. Yet the possibility exists within the church for a reinterpretation of family, as well as a sketch of what a church can look like when it attempts to understand itself as family which transcends the boundaries of natural and cherished blood relations. Prevailing cultural realities require the church to be a model of the spiritual family, with enough power to combat the disintegrating pressures which surround us both from within ourselves and without.

The healing church is one that knows what it means to be unconditionally liable for another simply because he or she is brother or sister in Christ. Such a family ultimately does not recognize the same limits that are established in the average Christian family as we know it. The family which is shaped around being called to be God's people does not love its natural family less, but it is always aware that it is living out of a different understanding, a different order. This order is rooted in not having to *deserve* God's steadfast love, but having, in the end, to choose the costly act of receiving that kind of love. That love requires of us the relinquishment of the controls of our *own* lives and our *own* families.

A third mark of the healing church is that it *belongs to another order*, and as such, travels lightly, in the understanding of being pilgrims in a strange land. Paradoxically, the church which has found its identity as the people of God is called to establish a new order and to live in it on this earth, rather than merely to anticipate the end of time in which that order will be revealed in all of its fullness.

A common misconception has occurred in many corners

of the church: individual salvation has become stressed to the exclusion of the knowledge that we are called to be the kingdom and to work for the kingdom now, on this earth, and not wait passively for the eschatological climax of history.

Knowing that we are a called people enables us to detach ourselves from our culture enough to see the spiritual realities which are frequently obliterated—perhaps most often by those who resist the fact that the road is narrow which leads to salvation. The way put before us by Christ and his committed followers throughout the decades has been costly. The challenge for the church, then, is to discover the pearl of great price and, as a called people, to obtain it.

The fourth mark of the healing church is that it is *on a pilgrimage in search of self-understanding, a pilgrimage toward mission*. The powerful connection between healing and mission is one that we in the church will have to learn to make. In Isaiah 6, the prophet's healing and vocational calling are simultaneous. The healing church has discovered this wisdom and gives its members a creative work to do as well as offering comfort for the troubled soul. This recognition of the *healing power of a beloved work* describes the fifth mark of the healing church.

The healing church recognizes the truth of Carl Jung's assertion that we must come to terms with our shadows in order to realize our creative potential. The church presents a picture of a people recuperating from the wounds of their personal histories, while at the same time responding to God's call to gird up their loins and do the work he has given them to do. Henri Nouwen set before us the image of the wounded healer. We in the church are wounded, and it is in the recognition of the depth of those wounds, and the recognition that we are called by God *in our wounded state* to do his work, that our true freedom comes.

The church must be that place where sin can be openly acknowledged and transformed by the love of Christ in the fellowship of the believers. If this is our choice, we must be prepared for what Paul Tournier has called "the painful path of humiliation which opens into the royal road of grace and freedom." Tournier reminds us that Jacob dared to wrestle with God, yet his soul and body were preserved. The other part of that story must be remembered as well, for it has important meaning for an understanding of the true cost of being the church. Jacob wrestled with the angel and God put his mark upon Jacob—he went away from the encounter limping. Jacob experienced the realities of his wounded self in his bond to be God's own. That, it seems, is our lot if we choose to undergo the costly way of seeing ourselves as we truly are and choosing to follow Christ at all costs.

The healing church is the church which knows its costly heritage and which, like the prodigal son, returns to claim the undeserved inheritance of the steadfast love of God. When the church returns to the Father's house, it will discover healing and reconciliation. Such is the experience of those within faith communities who have chosen the costly life for the sake of the joy that comes in the deep sharing of life with one another. In themselves, such communities are not sanctified or above reproach. But they make a statement about their choice—a choice to come apart from modern culture to cast their lot with God's people, in the conviction that this is the true path to freedom. The fruits of such a time in the life of God's people have been described in Isaiah 35:

The wilderness and the dry land shall be glad,
the desert shall rejoice and blossom;
like the crocus it shall blossom abundantly,
and rejoice with joy and singing. . . .

Then the eyes of the blind will be opened,
and the ears of the deaf unstopped;
then shall the lame man leap like a hart
and the tongue of the dumb sing for joy. . . .

but the redeemed shall walk there.
And the ransomed of the Lord shall return,
and come to Zion with singing;
everlasting joy shall be upon their heads;
they shall obtain joy and gladness,
and sorrow and sighing shall flee away.

The church that can choose the abundant life offered through costly discipleship is the church in whose midst healing flows until the very desert blossoms and is populated by a people who know that healing and salvation are one.

APPENDIX
New Hope for Health

Section I   How Do You Spell Wholistic?

This section presents a brief statement explaining the difference between church-related and general holistic approaches to health care.

Section II   Study Questions

These questions are intended for use in giving workshops in local congregations or for discussion groups wanting to use this book as a springboard for interest in the subject. Also included is a sample workshop format that was used with a midwestern church.

Section III   Stress Exercises

This assortment of exercises is designed to help individuals assess their own levels of stress, including the inventory used at participating Westberg clinics.

Section IV   Bibliography

This listing includes a specific focus on religion and health and other general readings in holistic health care as well as reviews of selected books and tapes on Divine healing.

SECTION I

For those who are confused by the term "holistic," the following short article may provide useful information.

How Do You Spell "Wholistic"?

Another prevention-oriented health movement, usually spelled "holistic" (but not always) has picked up ideas from Eastern religions, the occult, and various methods of healing often dismissed as quackery by the medical profession. The more Christian program of the Wholistic Health Care, Inc., may be confused with the more free-wheeling holistic experiments.

The holistic health movement has come into being for many of the same reasons as the Wholistic Movement. Both are concerned about escalating costs of health care (about 9 percent of the G. N. P. with 40 percent representing hospital bills) and inaccessibility or maldistribution of health care favoring the affluent urbanite. Illness that has been termed clinically iatrogenic (physician induced), which may be the result of unnecessary hospitalizations, surgery, or detrimental effects of prescription drugs, has paved the way for the growing popularity of both health movements which frequently criticize the mechanistic or disease-oriented approach to people that focuses exclusively on the physiological.

The Holistic Movement also builds on many of the same concepts as Wholistic Health Care, most notably those of stress prevention, and the importance of caring for the whole person.

In method and theology, however, the two movements are oceans apart, literally as well as figuratively.

While open to certain non-Western and nontraditional treatments such as acupuncture and biofeedback, the approach at the Wholistic Centers is basically traditional, keeping within the bounds of the standards set by the American Medical Association.

In contrast, the vast majority of Holistic Health treatments are nontraditional. Virtually nothing is excluded. The May issues of *New Age*, a leading Holistic journal, included articles and advertisements on hypnosis, acupuncture, tantric sexual rebirthing, est, Eselen, Shiatsu, yoga, polarity therapy, vegetarian cooking, and a feature article by Irving Oyle, M.D., who details ten steps for holistic health. By putting oneself into a hypnotic trance similar to the "unbounded awareness" phase of Transcendental Meditation, one can get in touch with one's spirit guide who will give helpful health counsel. The guide often takes the form of a creature, such as a lizard or coyote.

While not all of the holistic techniques are infused with a monistic or occult world-view, there is generally a high degree of metaphysical contamination in most articles written and seminars given by holistic health enthusiasts. Interviews with nurses and other health-related professionals have indicated that their involvement often leads them into some form of Eastern religion.

A written statement available to patients from the Wholistic Health Centers, Inc. promises that they will not try to moralize or convert people to any religion. Nonetheless, the underlying assumptions on which the movement is based are theistic. God is viewed as personal, transcendent, and involved in the world he has created. He is not, says Wholistic health care leader, Granger Westberg, "just a bowl of cosmic ether." An Eastern mediator whose idea of ideal health is to merge into the universal, impersonal "OM" is likely to be disappointed when he meets a pastoral counselor who suggests that meditating on the Bible may help to build a positive mature faith that can in turn help a person cope more realistically with the stress of life.

For a critique of the holistic (Eastern and occult version) health program, see the *Journal of the Spiritual Counterfeits Project*, August 1978 (or send a dollar to Box 4308, Berkeley, California 94704).

Sharon Fish, R.N.
Reprinted by permission of *Eternity* Magazine
© 1979 Evangelical Ministries, Inc.
1716 Spruce Street
Philadelphia, PA 19103

SECTION II

Sample of a Seminar on Holistic Health
in the Church's Life

In our first session, we looked at an overview of what was to
come during the following five weeks. We answered the question, what is church-related holistic health care and how is it
different from other medical treatment? We took an inventory of
Third's existing healing ministries using that term in the broadest sense and came up with a surprising variety—from *Stephen
ministers* to the luncheons for retirees. We noted that not much
has been organized around prayer for healing either in the form
of a specific service or in a prayer partner format.

We also began to discuss the theological basis for this approach to health care. Next we completed looking at the theological and Biblical justification for holistic health care in the
context of Jesus' ministry of healing persons, the disciples' emphasis on healing and the early church's practice of anointing
the sick. We also looked at two current models of church related
whole-person health care; Columbia Road Health Services in
inner city Washington, D.C. and the Vellore Christian Medical
College and Hospital in South India. We looked a little at what
goes into the formation of such a health service.

From there, the class focused on the pastoral aspect of this
type of health care. Particularly, we highlighted a discussion
revolving around faith and health. We looked at the stress factors involved in producing illness and the type of faith outlook
which is likely to promote wholeness even if it does not produce

freedom from disease. However, we recognized through the use of case studies how faith or lack of faith affects everything we do including our total health.

Tom Mansen, R.N., from the Hope/Calvin department of nursing spoke to us about the medical component of health and wholeness. He told of the role of stress in creating serious illnesses and listed some which are commonly referred to as "stress illnesses" such as heart disease, high blood pressure and strokes to name a few. Tom was involved in cardiology and intensive care nursing before coming to Hope.

The climax of our series was a presentation by a woman who told of her near-death encounter which led to four years of serious illness, a diagnosis of terminal illness, yet eventual recovery through utilizing a holistic approach. She worked with medical doctors and specialists, the pastors of her church, and with a gifted Christian psychologist to unlock the key to recovery. It was surprising to all of us the extent to which her entire immune system revolted until she uncovered the psychological and spiritual roots of her trouble.

When we asked where to go from all this input during the closing session, we focused attention on the already existing ministries at *Third*. We also discussed the role of prayer in the healing process. It was suggested that follow-up on the pastor implementing a prayer for healing service be explored. Interest in a more private format such as prayer partners was also stated. Another idea was to appoint a Minister of Health Care; another option would be to ask the minister of parish life to focus more on health-related concerns within the congregation and to coordinate all the related ministries in this area. Concern was expressed that pastoral care emphasize prayer with the sick, troubled or dying. A number of other resources for healing included high-quality Christian counseling, journaling, and support groups such as the *koinonea* groups.

For people who could not join us, I recommended reading a provocative new book called *Kicking Your Stress Habits* by Donald

Tubesing. This book contains concise helpful aids for dealing with stress and is certainly an easy to read starting place for personalizing what church-related whole-person health care offers. The paperback may be ordered for $10 from Whole Person Associates, P.O. Box 3151, Duluth, MN 55003.

A Parish Inventory

Let's begin with an inventory or analysis or diagnosis of the health and healing ministry within your parish.

A. First, privately list *who* is doing *what* in the area of health and healing in your parish.

_____

_____

_____

_____

_____

_____

_____

_____

B. Compile a common list of who is doing what at your parish. (Use newsprint if it is available.)

C. Once you have compiled the list, you may want to review what you see:
1. Is much happening?
2. Are many people or only a few involved? Are those involved "professionals"?
3. What's the quality of the work being done?
4. Are there gaps in the parish's health and healing activities? Is there "room" for improvement or expansion?

D. List here any thoughts or insights you have discovered about your parish's health and healing activity through this inventory.

_____

_____

Study Questions on In the Land of the Living

1. Whole-person health care is a return to the biblical view of persons as a unity of body, mind and spirit. Are you surprised that modern society abandoned the biblical view?

2. There are often spiritual roots to illness which include chiefly the lack of reconciliation to a significant other or God. Can you think of examples you would be willing to share?

3. Whole-person care is oriented toward health and wholeness rather than disease. It emphasizes each person's responsibility for their own life and health. How do you react to being told you are responsible for your health?

4. All types of healing were a dominant theme in Jesus' mission on earth. Since this is true, why doesn't the church follow Christ's example today?

5. Christ gave the church the gift of healing power to be used to strengthen its life. How might belief and acceptance of this gift change your congregational life?

6. Wholeness in Christ is true wholeness. It is an inner harmony, integration of the personality and a transparency before God and others. Can a person be considered whole in the midst of a terminal diagnosis?

7. What are your own assumptions about suffering?

8. What do you understand to be the role of confession in the healing process?

9. We are all called to be wounded healers. How do you feel about that statement? Can you be wounded and also heal?

10. Medicine and faith are complementary agents of healing but they are often pitted against each other. How do you view their connections?

11. Can you share an example of how faith enhances health?

12. Are you aware of aspects of religious belief which, when used negatively, have produced destructive influences on your health or on that of someone you know?

13. What is appropriate guilt? What is false guilt? How can you discover the difference?

14. Can you comment on the case histories we considered? Have you or someone you know ever shared similar experiences?

15. Is Helene's near death experience clear to you? Have you ever known someone who had this type of encounter with death but lived and learned something from it?

16. Is there anything in Helene's story that explains why she would have become so sick for so long aside from purely biological factors?

17. How does Helene interpret her experience in light of the interrelationship between stress and illness?

18. Does this story challenge you to search yourself for stress and faith related factors in your own health picture?

19. Does your church have a setting and commitment similar or dissimilar to that which spawned Columbia Road Health Services?

20. Would your church ever consider beginning a health service within its building or in another location?

21. How is the role of the pastoral care department at the Christian Medical College in Vellore, South India, different from other Christian hospitals?

22. Why would they be trying to use holistic health care in India when it is only used in a few hospitals in the U.S.?

23. Is there anything in these descriptions of church-related health ministries which challenges you in your own situation, both professionally and in terms of your local church?

A List of Topics for Church Study Groups

I. The Biblical Witness to Healing
   A. Healing is Jesus' ministry: Primary is his will to heal. Suffering Servant—with his stripes we are healed.
   B. Healing as a sign of the Kingdom of God; breaking in of the new order—restoring order out of the chaos which came about in the Fall.
   C. The Church and the gift of healing.
      1. Role of ministering persons—to be an enabler of persons in saying yes to life, both in illness and in health.
      2. The church is the mediator of healing in society today.
      3. The church's role in making the healing charism manifest in its midst; gift of healing given to the Body for the use of all.

II. Salvation and Healing
   A. It is not whether we are religious or non-religious but whether we are saying yes or no to life. How we use our faith determines how we will accept or reject our situation. Example of response to suffering.
   B. The root of Salvation is Salve = to heal, to become whole; we need to minister to the whole person. Salvation is what brings healing to the whole person.

III. God's Will
   A. Why did this happen to me/who is to blame?
   B. What is the meaning I can find in my situation?
   C. Divine providence/God's permissive will?

IV. Questions of meaning in illness and subsequent death
   A. What is ultimate: becoming whole or relationship with God?

B.   What is less than ultimate in my life? My health? Can I
be whole and be dying of cancer? Wholeness is a dynamic process of integration and harmony with
oneself, others and the Creator.
C.   Can I pray for healing? Judeo-Christian tradition
makes it clear that petitions for healing are part of a
life of faith. Healing can and does occur for some people, but there are no guarantees.
D.   Why doesn't God heal me or my loved one? Healing is
a mysterious gift of God. It does not come because we
court it. Just as it is clear that we can have faith and
hope for healing, it is clear that we must accept the
reality of what is given. Suffering and death do exist
side by side with divine intervention and healing. It
takes flexibility and hope to be able to live with this
kind of paradox.

Worksheet for a Philosophy of Christian Health Care

Developed by the Christian Community Health
Fellowship of the Voice of Calvary, Jackson, Mississippi

1. Why do we do Christian Health Care?
2. What is Christian Health Care? (What does *health* mean to you? How does our health care differ from the world's health care?)
3. How do we do Christian Health Care? (In what specific areas does Jesus' example affect our work? How does it direct us to do health care?)
4. What effect does Jesus' deep concern for the poor, so often expressed in the Gospels, have on the way we do health care?
5. What does the Gospel require in terms of nurturing (or breaking) our self images? How does this affect the way we relate to each other? the way we relate to patients?
6. What does the Gospel require of our life style? How does this differ from what the world expects of people in medicine?
7. What are some examples of Christian health care that flesh out a consistent philosophy of Christian community health?

SECTION III

This section is focused on increasing our awareness of the relationship between stress and illness. This collection of exercises is intended to encourage you to personalize your study of this subject and to discover firsthand how stress may be creating illness in your life.

The first exercise, a stress inventory prepared by Thomas Holmes of the University of Washington, may be used to simply acquaint you with the number of stressful events you have been carrying within the past year. As the author states, a score of over 300 may indicate that you are courting illness in the near future.

You will notice that the inventory includes both good stress and bad stress. For example, a promotion at work is generally a positive thing, even though it is stressful to adjust to a change of position. A death is obviously a negative form of stress. Our lives are filled with stress, and stress in itself is not bad for our health. It is a matter of how much prolonged stress we can manage creatively. This varies widely among individuals. When a person carries too much stress over a prolonged period of time without resolution, they are very likely to become ill.

"The Stress of Adjusting to Change" can be used to discover the total amount of stressful situations you are currently involved in. We don't usually stop to reflect on our total life picture, but doing this may help prevent overly stressful, illness-producing living.

The Stress of Adjusting to Change

Below are listed many of the events in life which have been found to produce individual stress reactions in a cross section study conducted by Dr. Thomas H. Holmes at the University of Washington. The scale value of each event reflects the amount of stress and disruption they cause in the life of the average person's life. More than 200 units accumulated during the period of a year can cause some individuals to exceed their stress tolerance with resulting physical and psychological reactions. Of course, individuals do vary in their tolerance for stress so that these figures should only be taken as a rough guide.

Of the people who scored 300 on the Holmes Survey, almost 80 percent got sick in the near future; of those who scored 150 to 299, about 50 percent got sick; and of those who scored less than 150, only 30 percent became sick.

Thus, the higher your score, the harder you should work to stay well.

EVENT	SCALE VALUE	YOUR SCORE
Death of spouse	100	
Divorce	73	
Marital separation	65	
Jail term	63	
Death of close family member	63	
Personal injury or illness	53	
Marriage	50	
Fired at work	47	
Marital reconciliation	45	
Retirement	45	
Change in health of family member	44	
Pregnancy	40	
Sex difficulties	39	
Gain of new family member	39	
Business readjustment	39	

Change in financial state	38	_____
Death of close friend	37	_____
Change to different line of work	36	_____
Increased arguing with spouse	35	_____
Mortgage over $10,000	31	_____
Foreclosure of mortgage or loan	30	_____
Change in responsibilities at work	29	_____
Son or daughter leaving home	29	_____
Trouble with in-laws	29	_____
Outstanding personal achievement	28	_____
Wife begins or stops work	26	_____
Begin or end school	26	_____
Change in living conditions	25	_____
Revision of personal habits	24	_____
Trouble with boss	23	_____
Change in work hours or conditions	20	_____
Change in residence	20	_____
Change in schools	20	_____
Change in recreation	19	_____
Change in church activities	19	_____
Change in social activities	18	_____
Mortgage or loan less than $10,000	17	_____
Change in sleeping habits	16	_____
Change in family reunions/get togethers	15	_____
Change in eating habits	15	_____
Vacation	13	_____
Christmas	12	_____
Minor violations of the law	11	_____

Your total _____
Reprinted in *New York Times*
June 10, 1973

Stress Buildup

This exercise gives an opportunity for you to assess your current use of energy and evaluate it. Just because we are expending energy in certain areas does not mean we feel good about it or have a sense of choice about it. This exercise gives a chance to look at how you are currently spending your time and to decide whether or not you want to make some changes. It also focuses on areas that tend to drain creative energy and gives an opportunity to assess choices there, too.

Sharing in small groups may facilitate a feeling of hopefulness as you discover that others, too, are struggling to set priorities and balance their individual needs with work-related needs and relational needs. By sharing your frustrations and hopes, you may find some new ways to organize your life and time that will ultimately be more satisfying.

Vocation is integrally related to health and wholeness. The following exercises may be helpful for both individuals or study groups in assessing current vocational involvement and future direction. It may also serve as a catalyst for churches considering what type of healing ministry they may wish to create.

First, go through the list and rate your present energy expenditure on a continuum of 1 to 3, with 3 being high and 1 being low.

Career	1	2	3
Friends	1	2	3
Socializing	1	2	3
Spouse/Significant other	1	2	3
Children	1	2	3
Sports	1	2	3
Hobbies	1	2	3
Self-Growth	1	2	3
Community Service	1	2	3
Personal Time	1	2	3
Spirituality	1	2	3
Adventure	1	2	3

Now, go through the list a second time and mark how you'd prefer to spend your energy. Next, check the activities on the following list that are sapping your energy.

_____ Time limits or deadlines
_____ Production limits
_____ Worry about relationships: family, relatives, boss, neighbors, co-workers, friends and church
_____ Worry about money and paying bills
_____ Worry about home repairs
_____ General work discomfort
_____ Understimulation and lack of challenge
_____ Disorder
_____ Competition for promotions, pay raises, praise
_____ Poor eating patterns
_____ Crowded physical space or poor facilities
_____ Other

The higher you score, the harder you should work to stay well.

Dick Leider and Janet Hagburg
The Inventurers

What Do You Hear the Lord Saying???

Recently the Franciscan Sisters of the Poor, embarked on a process to help each one of us look at our individual goals. Realizing that the Holy Spirit speaks to the whole body through the guidance He gives the individual, we sought to gather this wisdom through the sharing of our individual leadings with each other.

First Stage: Each of us received five questions which we were asked to examine in seven different areas or levels of our life.

Five Questions: (At X insert each of the seven levels, e.g. physical, emotional, etc.)

1.   What do I hear the Lord saying in Scripture with regard to my X growth this year?

2.   How do I hear the community (family) calling me X-ly this year?

3.   How do I want to grow X-ly this coming year?

4.   What am I willing to do in order for these X wants to become a reality?

5.   What of these X goals
     (a)   am I responsible for?
     (b)   do I want to share with a friend?
     (c)   do I want to share with my community (family)?

7 Levels:

Physical	Social
Emotional	Communal
Intellectual	Ministerial
Spiritual	

Second Stage: We shared what we had individually heard in response to these questions with a friend and/or local community, and experienced a deepening sense of support and encouragement both individually and corporately. A new strength and oneness resulted.

Third Stage: As the local communities (families) moved into "communal goal setting," there was a greater clarity and respect for the views of each individual as she searched the following questions:

1. From what we have heard from the individual directions, how do we as a local community (family) want to grow this year?
2. What do we want to do? Is this realistic?
3. What are we willing to do?
4. How will we do this? Who will be responsible?

You might want to try a similar process of sharing, caring, and growing as a family or community by prayerfully sharing your individual goals with each other.

Quarterly, *Living Water*, 1979, Fall, Vol. 2, #4, Newsletter of the Institute for Christian Healing.

Betty Igo, F.S.P.

Personal Health Inventory

The final exercise is the "Personal Health Inventory" designed for use in a church-related wholistic health center. We used this inventory with our clients at Columbia Road Health Services. It was designed by the staff of Wholistic Health Centers Inc. in Hinsdale, Illinois.

As you fill out this inventory, just as you would as a client in a wholistic health care center, you may find that you would like your own family doctor or specialist to read through it because of the additional information it gives about you.

Welcome to the Wholistic Health Center.

Our intention in your first visit is to engage you in an individualized plan for becoming and staying healthy. We believe that being healthy is more than having a body that works well; it is feeling good about yourself, dealing creatively with the people and situations around you, and growing spiritually toward a sense of wholeness.

In our initial planning conference you will meet with a health care team consisting of a physician, nurse, and director of counseling. We'll talk together about which of our professional skills would be most helpful to you and arrive at a plan for working together. We recognize that the final decisions about the plan are up to you; the best we can do is make recommendations and offer our services.

We've found that people appreciate and benefit from an opportunity to reflect on all of their concerns prior to the initial conference. This pamphlet is offered as a tool to help focus your reflections before the planning conference. Please bring it with you.

If you have any questions about this pamphlet or the conference, please ask any of the staff. We appreciate your comments.

Your Name: _____Date: _____

LIFE EVENT CHECKLIST

Check events which have occurred in the past few years and circle those that have been most important to you. Reflect on these changes before completing the remainder of the inventory.

The Spiritual Dimension

_____ Change in relationship with God
_____ Change in Church activity or prayer life
_____ Significant spiritual experience
_____ Spiritual emptiness
_____ Constant feelings of guilt or anxiety
Other: _____

Personal Events/Changes

_____ Death of a close friend or family member
_____ Personal injury, illness or hospitalization
_____ Pregnancy (Or pregnancy of spouse)
_____ Loss of self confidence
_____ Outstanding achievement (graduation, promotion)
_____ Change in eating habits
_____ Change in sexual activity
_____ Change in sleeping patterns
_____ Change in energy level
_____ Considered suicide
_____ Change in religious belief or practice
_____ Stress related to vacation
_____ Change in relationship with parents
_____ Change in recreational time/activity
_____ Trouble with the law
_____ Change in time schedule
Change in _____ drinking _____ smoking _____ drug use
Other: _____

Marital Relationship

_____ Married _____ Divorced _____ Separated
_____ Widowed _____ Living together
_____ Disagreements over money management
_____ Increased emotional distance
_____ Trouble with in-laws
_____ Spouse beginning or stopping work or school
Other: _____

Household Events

_____ Family member left home
_____ Gain of a new member (birth, parents moving in, adoption, etc.)
_____ Spouse at home more than before
_____ Problems with children at home
_____ Change in residence
_____ Remodeling or building
_____ Change in health/behavior/attitude of a member of the household
_____ Change in neighbors or neighborhood
Other: _____

Vocational Events

_____ New Job, or new line of work
_____ Quit _____ Fired _____ Retired _____ Laid Off
_____ Less job security
_____ Promotion _____ Demotion
_____ Trouble with work associates
_____ Change in hours, conditions, travel, etc.
Other: _____

Financial Changes

_____ Changes in financial state (better or worse)
_____ Major mortgage or loan taken over
_____ Foreclosure of mortgage or loan
Other: _____

1. Physical symptoms I'm concerned about:

_____

_____

_____

2. Feelings/emotions I'm concerned about:

_____

_____

_____

3. Goals toward which I'd like to begin moving:

_____

_____

_____

4. My strong points and special abilities moving toward my goals:

_____

_____

_____

5. Kinds of help I need in moving toward my goals:

_____

_____

_____

SECTION IV

What About Divine Healing?
(A Book Survey)

Nothing concerns people more than their health or that of those close to them. In the past five years a whole library of books has appeared on the subject of healing and the problem of pain, which is the reverse of the health coin. The following discussion samples what is currently available. The books reflect different perspectives and traditions. Many of them are written by charismatics, where the renewed interest in healing began, though such mainline denominations as the Reformed and Methodist churches are also represented.

Sooner or later suffering finds us all. Whether we respond with prayers for healing or prayers for acceptance, we can find comfort and guidance in the experiences of Christians who have grappled with these issues. Most of these books have helped me. I include some books that aren't useful to show the differences in quality of books on healing. And I look at three books that raise the obvious question, What if you aren't healed? I want to show the reader how to evaluate books on healing so they can find the best books available. The place to begin is with Morton Kelsey's study *Healing and Christianity: In Ancient Thought and Modern Times* (Harper & Row). Kelsey to date has written the most complete work, theologically and historically, on healing. Kelsey says that "this is not a book on the method of practice of religious healing. Instead it is an attempt to provide a theological foundation, based on historical and scientific understanding, for a serious ministry of healing today."

Kelsey's book, based on charismatic theology, represents a radical departure from the mainstream of modern theological thought on the matter of divine healing. It is a comprehensive history of sacramental healing in the Christian church from biblical times to the present. A theme that runs through charismatic literature on the subject of healing is the belief that it is God's ordinary will to heal, and that such healing comes primarily through supernatural intervention.

The best writers on the subject argue that healing was a primary ministry of Jesus and his church, but that it fell into disrepute sometime during the Middle Ages, when the sacrament of anointing the sick became relegated to a rite for the dying. Kelsey makes a strong case for returning a concern for healing to the ordinary life of a congregation and demystifying the experience of being healed by God of one's infirmities, be they emotional or physical, congenital or accidental. Kelsey, an Episcopal rector, researched his study for fifteen years and has had far more than an academic relationship to the subject of healing. As he puts it, "I have seen the things of which I write." I believe him.

For a person who wants a more pragmatic book on healing, Francis MacNutt has written one. Father MacNutt, like Kelsey, is a theologian in the charismatic renewal movement who has been involved in a healing ministry for about ten years. *Healing* (Ave Maria) is an excellent book. It contains detailed information on the charismatic healing style, which has spread across the world in the years since Vatican II. MacNutt describes how he was drawn into a healing ministry and responds directly to questions concerning why some people are not healed. MacNutt's maturation is reflected in the contrast between his first and second books. *The Power to Heal* (Ave Maria) enjoys more subtlety and open admission of the mystery of God's ways regarding why some persons' prayers for healing are answered affirmatively and some negatively.

I do not find in MacNutt, however, a satisfactory treatment of the theology of suffering or of the cross, which is the critical question to be resolved in the matter of divine healing. Why does God apparently heal some people and not others? Can suffering be redemptive? But in *The Power to Heal*, MacNutt is far more direct than in *Healing*, his earlier work. He admits that he doesn't know the answers. Readers searching for books on healing written with balance and maturity can anticipate being challenged by MacNutt's clear and forthright message: healing power is available to everyone—healing is the birthright of the Christian church. But MacNutt does not hit you over the head; he invites you to test it for yourself.

Being the sister of the current president makes it difficult for her work to be accepted in its own right, but Ruth Carter Stapleton's message is worth hearing. In her two books, *The Gift of Inner Healing* and *The Experience of Inner Healing* (Word), she shares simply and directly her insight on the nature of emotional healing. Like MacNutt, she shows decided growth between books.

If it's a question of reading only one, make it the second in which she shares her own experience of inner healing. She conveys a spirit of warmth and hope throughout the book that will thaw the most cynical reader.

Stapleton has a gift to share with us: the repression and denial of one's true feelings is the antithesis of Christianity and can only lead to spiritual, often physical, death. If this sounds like pop psychology à la the Sensitivity Group Movement's cheap grace variety, it is not. She demonstrates repeatedly in both books what Paul Tournier expressed in *Guilt and Grace:* The painful path of sin and humiliation precedes the royal road of grace and forgiveness. Inner healing is not a cheap idea. It means tough repentance and restitution.

The refreshing thing about Stapleton is that she is convinced that Christ loves and forgives the feelings of the inner child each of us has, and that through prayer and "faith imagination" the painful memories that still dominate our present thoughts, activities, and relationships can be healed by him. Along with Kelsey and MacNutt, Stapleton respects the insights of modern psychology and acknowledges their usefulness. A mark of maturity on charismatic literature on healing is its respect of medical science.

The most significant theological aspect of charismatic literature on healing is the conviction that sickness is evil and inconsistent with the intention of God toward the creation. Sickness is the direct result of the Fall; salvation brings wholeness and health if we but ask through prayer. The healing miracles of Jesus and the disciples is a sign of the Kingdom of God.

Healing Life's Hurts: Healing Memories Through the Five Stages of Forgiveness (Paulist) written by two brothers, both Catholic priests, is a major addition to the work done by Stapleton on healing the emotions. The Linn brothers have used the Kübler-Ross stages of death and dying to express the process for healing memories and emotions. As they put it, healing a memory is like dying. Therefore, they take us through the five stages of forgiveness: denial, anger, bargaining, depression, and acceptance, and illustrate through personal experience and examples how to uncover and forgive the hurts that have occurred over the course of a lifetime. *Healing Life's Hurts* combines theory with practice, and includes several exercises on how a person may guide him or herself through the process of forgiveness, which is necessary to healing. This is an important companion to Stapleton's work because it is designed for use by small groups to help build the church's life.

The Linn brothers, with the help of Barbara Shlemon, a registered nurse with whom they have shared a healing ministry, have written another book on healing. *To Heal as Jesus Healed* (Ave Maria) explores in the light of their own experiences in a ministry of healing the rite of anointing the sick. The authors provide numerous examples of healings and demonstrate that the new Roman Catholic Rite of Anointing is in keeping with the original place of healing in the ministry of Jesus and the life of the early church. This book offers limited usefulness, because of its focus on the Roman tradition, rather than on the scriptural basis for healing.

Althouse, in his *Rediscovering the Gift of Healing* (Abingdon), is involved in a ministry of healing primarily in the United Methodist Church. He relies heavily on MacNutt and Kelsey to build his historical and theological basis for healing as an ordinary mission in the church's life. The brief study includes suggestions on how to begin a healing ministry in one's local church.

In contrast, George Bennet, former hospital chaplain, working in the church healing ministry trust of the Church of England, has written a refreshing and brief account of his experiences with and belief in healing as an ordinary part of the church's life in *In His Healing Steps* (Judson). Anglican and Roman Catholic charismatics who come from traditions steeped in the sacraments seem to maintain a more balanced and mature relationship to the gifts of the Holy Spirit and decisions about their place in the life of the larger church. Bennet is a clear example of this pastoral maturity. He does not see healing in black-and-white simplicity, and is not afraid to discuss why some are not healed after fervent prayer. Nor does he explain this by telling us that they did not have enough faith.

Bennet maintains that the very name of Jesus implies healing: It means God saves or God heals, that it is the nature of Jesus to heal, that where the presence of Christ is there is healing. He speaks about the power of the principalities that lie beneath all our disease, and that in most sickness there is some malignancy that is buried even from conscious awareness that needs attending. His book is not history or theology but a testimony of the power of a healed and reconciled relationship with God.

George Martin's *Healing: Reflections on the Gospel* (Servant) attempts a short interpretation of some of the biblical material concerning healing. It is too brief to be definitive and although it is well written, it lacks depth. One would do better to read Kelsey and MacNutt for a more integrated analysis of the relationship of the biblical case for healing to the present implications for a healing ministry in the church's life.

Two books that I would not recommend are both from the

Gospel Publishing House of the Assemblies of God. *The Case for Divine Healing* by Bill Popejoy and *By His Stripes: A Biblical Study on Divine Healing* by Hugh Jeter are characteristic of the over-simplification of which charismatics are often accused. They are glib and preachy. Although I do not doubt the sincerity of either individual regarding their convictions about divine healing and its usefulness to the church, the tone of these books makes true dialogue impossible. They are monologues, love affairs with their own convictions. Kelsey, MacNutt, Stapleton, and Bennet do not try to convert the reader. They believe the healing power of Christ will persuade and speak for itself. Popejoy builds his case for healing in an authoritarian, catechetical style, which is lifeless and unconvincing. He is out to prove it to us through the authority vested in Scripture.

By His Stripes, too, tries to build an airtight biblical case to sanction the practice of supernatural healing in the life of the Church. But the approach is brittle: isolated proof-texting of quotations from Scripture and the discouragement of honest doubt. If Christ included Thomas in his inner circle, so should Jeter in a matter as complex as the question of God's will in regard to sickness and suffering.

Healing is not a new thing for Roman Catholics and Anglicans; you sense immediately a maturity and an enthusiasm tempered by experience in the books they write. Reginald East, an Anglican priest, has written a short study *Heal the Sick* (Dimension). His aim is to encourage Christians to accept a healing ministry as ordinary rather than pointing to it as something extraordinary. East wants to demonstrate that any Christian can enter into a healing ministry through prayer and openness to God's spirit. He offers clear and simple instruction to readers who are interested in learning to pray with others for healing. East shares his own initial reluctance to enter this kind of ministry; yet he felt directed to it by God's spirit. He discusses both physical and emotional healing and offers practical instruction for each type of prayer. This book will be of particular use to readers who are already convinced of the need for healing prayer and are seeking guidelines as they begin to practice it.

John Sanford, Episcopal priest and Jungian analyst, has written what is to me the most provocative study on healing of the books surveyed here. *Healing and Wholeness* (Paulist) relies on the work of psychologist Carl Jung for its arguments. Evangelicals who will note his somewhat unorthodox use of Scripture and the use he makes of wisdom from other religious traditions may distrust the book. Nonetheless, this refreshing and stimulating study suggests that the cultural definition of health as adjustment and adaptation is a false one, which needs revision. To illustrate his point he reminds the reader that in Nazi Germany the whole society was sick and that those who could not adjust or adapt to Hitler's views were not sick but profoundly well. Thus we need to reexamine our notion of wholeness.

Sanford suggests that one of the goals of life is a journey toward wholeness or individuation in Jungian terms. Sanford believes that the journey toward healing and wholeness cannot be equated with peace of mind. And that is encouraging. For Sanford, suffering is a real part of becoming whole. This is a book for the serious reader on the subject of healing. It emphasizes the philosophical and theological rather than the practical ways to find healing. Ironically, it may offer us more than many "how to" books because of the thinking it provokes.

The reader always returns to the question of suffering—whether in the celebrated account of Paul's thorn in the flesh, the story of Job, or the countless other examples in Scripture that imply that illness and suffering are sent from God, the author of all life. You cannot ignore the possibility that illness and suffering may serve a purpose in the lives of individuals. God's thoughts and ways are not ours. It is to this side of the question of healing that we must turn sooner or later, for it is painfully obvious to even the most zealous advocate of spiritual healing that everyone who prays is not healed.

Burton Seavey's *Why Doesn't God Heal Me?* (Creation) is a negative example; it represents many books that take the approach that the reason God doesn't heal us is that we don't have enough faith and are not obeying God's set of conditions for healing. This simplistic reduction of the mystery surrounding suffering will be of little use to the person who has prayed fervently and who has not received the healing he desires. What it will do is create guilt and feelings of failure. Seavey declares that "it is God's will to heal every born-again believer, when the conditions are met." Others who address the problem of pain concur that this thinking is not only bad theology but harms individuals who are looking for answers as to why they are not healed.

Here are two fine books that deal more adequately with the magnitude of suffering. Philip Yancey, former editor of *Campus Life,* says that pain has the potential for blessing in *Where Is God When It Hurts?* (Zondervan). He does this in fresh ways. He visits a leprosarium in Louisiana and discovers that those afflicted with leprosy do not have the built-in warning system in their nerve endings to warn them of danger. They lack the ability to feel pain. Pain, he says, is God's blessing that nobody wants. He raises the question of why there is such a thing as pain and of how people respond to pain. He suggests ways to cope with pain. He interviews Brian Sternberg and Joni Eareckson, two Christians whose lives were changed in split seconds to life-long quadraplegics. Brian and his family believe and hope for a complete healing miracle. Joni seeks to find meaning in the acceptance of her situation. Although prayer for healing is an option for Yancey, it fails to erase the problem of pain, since each of us must face death. Yancey wants to help those people trapped in pain to find meaning in and acceptance of their situation.

Robert Wise embraces the possibility of spiritual, even miraculous, healing, but he also grapples with the fact that all people who pray for healing are not healed. *When There Is No Miracle* (Regal) does this well. Wise writes as one who has believed in and experienced miracles.

"You ought to believe and anticipate the extraordinary inter-vening power of God, but God does not move at the snap of anyone's fingers, nor by the quoting of Scripture verses out of context. It is possible that you are missing the greatest miracle: that His sovereign hand is moving through every single event of your life whether the moment is exalted and exhilarating or tempestuous and traumatic."

Wise challenges us to anticipate God's work in our lives even when we see no concrete evidence of this, and when we experience only pain and frustration. He points out that the question, "Why did this happen to me?" needs to be transformed into "what is the intended meaning of this event?"

A member of the Reformed Church in America, Wise accepts a theology of providence based on the assumption that nothing is lost to God. No person or no moment of our existence is without meaning, though there will be many times when the present meaning will not be accessible to our understanding. Each chapter of *When There Is No Miracle* begins with an imaginary dialogue between the author and Jesus discussing a different aspect of pain and suffering. And each chapter closes with questions for discussing the convictions Wise expresses.

Ultimately, there should be no conflict in accepting the paradox that suffering exists side by side with supernatural healing; that the faith and hope to pray for healing is not fundamentally opposed to that faith and hope which accepts what is given, while looking to the transforming power of God's love.

Books on healing and suffering bring us to the basic question of human existence, the question of God's will. Although that will may remain ultimately a mystery, there are some aspects that are clear: God's will is dynamic, not static, and it always calls the Christian to greater faith and hope. Regardless of the outcome of individual suffering, our primary call is to be drawn deeper into relationship to him.

Karin Granberg-Michaelson
© 1978 *Christianity Today*, used by permission.

The Healing Ministry, by Francis MacNutt. Servant, 1976, five cassettes, $29.95.

These six talks were designed for use as a training course for individuals, prayer groups, and parishes seeking instruction on how to pray for healing. MacNutt has authored two books on healing: *Healing* and *The Power to Heal.* If you have read them, do not expect to discover a wealth of new material in these tapes. Perhaps the strongest aspect of the cassette series is that it powerfully proclaims the old, old story of Jesus and his love. Through a variety of techniques, from outlining kinds and characteristics of healing, through using personal experiences from his own healing ministry and that of others, to facilitate a healing service at a conference, MacNutt shares his vibrant belief in the healing power of Christ.

The first talk, "Four Kinds of Healing," outlines *spiritual, emotional, physical,* and *deliverance from evil spirits* as the major areas of healing. MacNutt makes the point that people cannot love through will power. It is useless to tell people they should love each other and form community because they cannot do it without the healing power of Christ which frees them from the hurts that bind them. MacNutt reinforces what persons involved in "whole person" health care see daily: that 80 to 90 percent of the patients doctors see are suffering from psychosomatic and psychogenic illnesses (that is, spiritual and psychological unrest produces physical symptoms). We are sick because of our inability to love and because we have not been loved.

"Problems in the Healing Ministry," tape two, reflects a maturing process that is taking place within MacNutt and others in the charismatic healing ministries. It directly addresses the problems that occur when people are not healed. MacNutt does not believe that God wants to heal everyone at once. He does believe that prayer for healing usually results in some improvement and doesn't ordinarily cause harm. The major concern he expresses is that there must be improved pastoral care for those who experience guilt because they have prayed or been prayed for and have not been healed. These people need to know God's love.

MacNutt uses the story of a young couple under the pastoral care of Graham Pulkingham. The woman had terminal cancer and was caught in a conflict between those who believed that God wished to heal her and those who felt it was her time to die. Pulkingham had a clear sense that prayer for healing was not God's will and counseled the couple accordingly. MacNutt shares the story to illustrate the importance of seeking to know the mind of Christ when we pray for healing.

In the third talk, "Inner Healing," MacNutt explains that as "children" we have as great a need for love as for food. Every experience is recorded in us like the growth rings on trees. Although psychology has given us a means of unearthing and bringing to light those things which torment us, it doesn't have the power to heal. MacNutt finds that through prayer, Christ can reenter our experiences and heal them.

"The Power of Persistent Prayer" is based on discoveries that MacNutt has made since the writing of his last book. He gives the example of Jesus healing the blind man who initially saw people as moving trees; praying a second time completed the healing. MacNutt has learned that some healings require repeated prayer over hours, days, months, and years. Other times, people are overcome by the Spirit and healed instantly, in the case of the apostle Paul's healing conversion. (His blindness required prayer at a later encounter.) Laying hands on the one who is receiving prayer, as well as praying in tongues, may facilitate healing, MacNutt believes. Praying in tongues, he says, can operate as a release when we do not know how to pray, and as a deeper form of abandonment to God's Spirit than our words and thoughts about what a person needs. MacNutt believes that we can pray for ourselves daily and expect to see more healing enter our lives.

In the fifth talk, "Healing and the Power of God," MacNutt reiterates the need for the church to be involved in a healing ministry. He believes that Jesus is the one who saves and heals.

We who seek healing for ourselves and others must be in submission to God in Christ as we pray. Our task is to listen and identify where and how God wants to use us as we pray. Mac-Nutt believes that ordinary Christians can pray for healing because of the power of God's Spirit that lives in us.

Finally, in "A Simple Way to Pray," we experience the speaker as he leads a healing service for 8,000 people and a television audience. This is MacNutt at his most compelling: as teacher and practitioner. The qualities that convince us are the fruits of the Spirit so evident in his humor, compassion, and down-to-earth simplicity.

Several things strike me about this fine series of tapes: the power of the human voice to communicate feelings in ways that the written word cannot; the fact that Servant asks you not to reproduce the tapes for commercial purposes, but encourages you to reproduce them for friends; and maybe most of all, Mac-Nutt's powerful reminders of God's love for us—a love that cuts into our darkness like a surgeon's scalpel and radiates the white-hot flame of healing throughout us. As the songwriter wrote: "The flame shall not hurt thee, I only design/ thy dross to consume and thy gold to refine." Francis MacNutt's greatest contribution may be his ability to arouse a renewed hunger both to know God's love and to share it with those we have never learned how to love.

Karin Granberg-Michaelson
Reprinted by permission of
Radix magazine
P.O. Box 4307
Berkeley, CA 94704

The Church's Healing Ministry

Blackburn, Lawrence H. "Spiritual Healing." *Journal of Religion and Health* (Vol. 15, No. 1, 1976): 34–37.

Boggs, Wade H., Jr. *Faith Healing and the Christian Faith,* Richmond, Virginia: John Knox Press, 1956.

Clinebell, Howard J., ed. *Community Mental Health: The Role of Church and Temple.* Nashville: Abingdon Press, 1970.

Doniger, Simon, ed. *Healing: Human and Divine: Man's Search for Health and Wholeness Through Science, Faith and Prayer.* New York: Association Press, 1957.

Frankl, Victor. *Man's Search for Meaning.* Boston: Beacon Press, 1963.

Johnson, Paul Emanuel. *Psychology of Pastoral Care.* Nashville: Abingdon-Cokesbury Press, 1953.

Kelsey, Morton T. *Healing and Christianity: In Ancient Thought and Modern Times.* New York: Harper and Row, Publishers, 1973.

Lambourne, R. A. *Community, Church and Healing.* London: Darton, Longman and Todd, Ltd., 1963.

MacNutt, Francis, O. P. *Healing.* Notre Dame: Ave Maria Press, 1974.

Niebuhr, Richard. *The Purpose of the Church and its Ministry.* New York: Harper and Brothers, 1956.

Oursler, Will. *The Healing Power of Faith.* New York: Hawthorne Books, Inc., 1957.

Rubenstein, Richard L. *After Auschwitz.* Indianapolis: Bobbs-Merrill, 1966.

Sharlemann, Martin H. "Toward a Theology of Healing," unpublished paper, Concordia Seminary, St. Louis, Mo.

Soelle, Dorothee. *Suffering.* Philadelphia: Fortress Press, 1975.

Suenens, Cardinal L. J. *A New Pentecost?* New York: Seabury Press, 1975.

Tillich, Paul. *The Courage to Be.* New Haven: Yale University Press, 1963.

Psychology and Religion

Bower, Robert K., ed. *Biblical and Psychological Perspectives for Christian Counselors*, Publishers Services, 1974.

Curran, Charles A. *Religious Values in Counseling and Psychotherapy*. New York: Sheed and Ward, 1969.

Colston, Lowell G., and Johnson, Paul E. *Personality and Christian Faith*. Nashville, Tennessee: Abingdon Press, 1972.

Dwyer, Walter W. *The Churches' Handbook for Spiritual Healing*. New York: Ascension Press, 1958.

Friedman, Maurine. "Healing through Meeting: A Dialogical Approach to Psychotherapy and Family Therapy," cited in *Psychiatry and the Humanities*, Vol. I, Joseph H. Smith, editor. New Haven: Yale University Press, 1976.

Fromm, Erich. *Psychoanalysis and Religion*. New Haven: Yale University Press, 1950.

Hanna, Charles Bartruff. *The Face of the Deep: The Religious Ideas of C. G. Jung*. Philadelphia: Westminster Press, 1967.

Hiltner, Seward. *Religion and Health*. New York: The Macmillan Company, 1943.

James, William. *The Varieties of Religious Experience: A Study in Human Nature*. New York: Modern Library, 1902.

Jung, Carl Gustav. *Psychology and Religion*. New Haven: Yale University Press, 1938.

Mowrer, O. Hobart. "Abnormal Reactions or Actions?" Dubuque, Iowa: Wm. C. Brown Company Publishers, 1966.

_____. *The New Group Therapy*. Insight Book. New York: Van Nostrand Reinhold Company, 1964.

Nouwen, Henri, J. M. *The Wounded Healer: Ministry in Contemporary Society*. Garden City, New York: Doubleday and Company, Inc., 1972.

Oates, Wayne E. *When Religion Gets Sick*. Philadelphia: The Westminster Press, 1970.

_____. *The Psychology of Religion*. Waco, Texas: Word Books, 1973.

150   In the Land of the Living

Oden, Thomas C. *Kerygma and Counseling: Toward a Covenant Ontology for Secular Psychotherapy.* Philadelphia: The Westminster Press, 1966.

Outler, Albert C. *Psychotherapy and the Christian Message.* New York: Harper and Brothers, Publishers, 1954.

Reeves, Robert B., Jr. "Healing and Salvation: Some Research and its Implications," Unpublished paper.

Tournier, Paul. *A Doctor's Casebook in Light of the Bible,* trans. by Edwin Hudson. London: SCM Press, 1954.

_____. *The Meaning of Persons,* trans. by Edwin Hudson. New York: Harper and Brothers, 1957.

_____. *Guilt and Grace: A Psychological Study,* trans. by Arthur W. Heathcote, J. J. Henry, and P. J. Allcock. New York: Harper & Row Publishers, 1962.

_____. *The Healing of Persons,* trans. by Edwin Hudson. New York: Harper and Row, 1965.

_____. *The Whole Person in a Broken World.* Harper & Row Publishers, 1981.

Tyrrell, Bernard J. *Christotherapy: Healing Through Enlightenment.* New York: Seabury Press, 1975.

Van Deusen, Dayton G. *Redemptive Counseling: Relating Psychotherapy to the Personal Meanings in Redemption.* Richmond, Virginia: John Knox Press, 1960.

Weatherhead, Leslie D. *Psychology, Religion and Healing.* Nashville: Abingdon Press, 1951.

Healing in Christian Community

Bonhoeffer, Dietrich. *Life Together,* trans. and intro. by John W. Doberstein. New York: Harper and Row, 1954.

Cosby, Gordon. *Handbook for Mission Groups.* Waco, Texas: Word Books, 1975.

Harper, Michael. *A New Way of Living: How the Church of the Redeemer, Houston, Found a New Life-style.* Plainfield, N.J.: Logos International, 1973.

Nouwen, Henri J. M. *Reaching Out: The Three Movements of the*

Spiritual Life. Garden City, New York: Doubleday and Company, Inc., 1975.

O'Connor, Elizabeth. *Call to Commitment.* New York: Harper and Row, 1963.

_____. *Journey Inward, Journey Outward.* New York: Harper and Row, 1971.

_____. *Eighth Day of Creation.* Waco, Texas: Word Publishers, 1971.

_____. *Search for Silence.* Waco, Texas: Word Publishers, 1972.

_____. *Our Many Selves.* New York: Harper and Row, 1971.

_____. *The New Community.* New York: Harper and Row, 1976.

_____. *Letters to Scattered Pilgrims.* New York: Harper and Row, 1982.

Pulkingham, W. Graham. *Gathered for Power.* Plainfield, N.J.: Logos Books, 1972.

_____. *They Left Their Nets: A Vision for Community Ministry.* New York: Morehouse-Barlow, Co., 1973.

Vanier, Jean. *Community and Growth,* trans. by Ann Shearer. Ramsey, N.J.: Paulist Press, 1979.

Annotated Bibliography for Wholistic Health Centers

Books in this bibliography are chosen for their characteristics as sources for further investigation and as seminal works for the model of wholistic health developed in the centers associated with Wholistic Health Centers, Inc.

Professional Approaches to Care

Fish, Sharon and Shelly, Judith. *Spiritual Care: The Nurse's Role.* Downers Grove, Ill.: Inter-Varsity Press, 1978.

A practical and conceptual guide for nurses in communicating with patients about the spiritual dimensions of their lives.

Concepts are not limited to nursing; ministers can learn from this book also.

Jourard, Sidney. *The Transparent Self*. Van Nostrand Reinhold, 1971.

I wish Jourard could update this book, because it's still the best starting point for professionals who don't know the values of self-disclosure when its's appropriate. Use in training of volunteers and staff. Ruel Howe's *The Miracle of Dialogue* is also basic. Both can give depth to many materials and workshops on communications.

Kaslof, Leslie, et al. *Wholistic Dimensions in Healing*. Garden City, N.Y.: Doubleday, 1978.

A comprehensive survey of the wholistic movement with brief essays by key figures and specific centers/projects who are currently working. Leans toward alternative forms of healing.

Moody, Raymond A. *Laugh After Laugh*. Jacksonville, Fla.: Headwaters Press, 1978.

". . . Humor works by rallying and being a manifestation of the will to live," says Moody, a physician/philosopher who also wrote *Life After Life*. A readable and scholarly work on the necessity of humor in health care. Good followup to Norman Cousins' articles in Saturday Review and New England Journal of Medicine about laughing himself back to health. Did you hear the one about . . .

Murray, Ruth and Zentner, Judith. *Nursing Concepts for Health Promotion*. N.J.: Prentice-Hall, 1979.

Principles and methods for nurses' involvement in encouraging healthy attitudes and behaviors. Used as a text in some nursing schools. Full of specific suggestions and examples. Large bibliographies.

Peterson, William M., et al. *The Process of Engagement*. Wholistic Health Centers, Inc., 1974.

A description of the principles and practice of engaging a person in the process of wholistic health care. Describes the health planning conference and alternative methods of engagement.

Rubin, Irwin M., et al. *Improving the Coordination of Care.* Cambridge, Mass.: Ballinger, 1975.

A workbook for a 7-week program for health teams. Well thought out and tested. You need a copy for each team member.

Somers, Anne R. *Promoting Health: Consumer Education and National Policy.* Germantown, Md.: Aspen Systems, 1976.

A survey of federal government policies to health promotion, and a who's who in government in this area. Not for those who want specific information, but a good feel of the policy positions. Anne Somers is active in several areas of health promotion.

Wise, Harold, et al. *Making Health Teams Work.* Cambridge, Mass.: Ballinger, 1974.

An expanded case study of the experience of an inner-city clinic. Good for team work in the medical model. Useful bibliographies. Comes in second to *Improving the Coordination of Care.*

The Health Care Scene Today

Dubos, Rene. *The Miracle of Health.* Harper and Row, 1979.

This and several other of Dubos' writings emphasize our relationship to health in the context of the human and physical environment. Following with *So Human an Animal.* Dubos is a microbiologist/pathologist/wholistic philosopher; one of a kind. Good companion to Lewis Thomas' *Lives of a Cell.*

Illich, Ivan. *Medical Nemesis.* Pantheon, 1982.

This social critic/prophet focuses his attention on American/Western medicine and points out the problems, primarily Iatrogenesis (the generation of disease by medicine itself). Has since been followed by Rick Carlson's *The End of Medicine* (more data, more visionary) and Robert Mendelsohn's *Confession of a Medical Heretic* (more scary).

Maxmen, Jerrold S. *The Post-Physician Era: Medicine in the 21st Century.* N.Y.: Wiley, 1976.

Futuristic look at medicine, very well laid out as a scenario in which physicians become administrators, teachers and specialists; specializing and pricing themselves out of direct service. Not a judgemental approach. Maxmen is a psychiatrist/writer at Albert Einstein School of Medicine.

Menninger, Carl. *The Vital Balance.* N.Y.: Viking Press, 1963.

Back in the early 60's, Menninger was saying that we don't know much about disease or health, except as pathology. He re-introduced the concept of balance as health. Following up with his 1973 book, *What Ever Became of Sin?*, an interesting challenge to the non-judgemental society and its detrimental effects.

Rogers, David E. *American Medicine: Challenge for the 1980s.* Cambridge, Mass.: Ballinger, 1978.

Rogers (son of Carl) is the physician/president of the Robert Wood Johnson Foundation. He shows signs of hope in medicine in the last ten years and points out areas still in need of attention, including ambulatory care, regionalized high technology, access for certain groups (poor children, elderly and handicapped) and improving the "texture" of interaction. Not a radical voice, but probably pointing the way that medicine (and funding) will really go in this decade.

Sobel, David E. *Ways of Health.* Harcourt Brace Jovanovich, 1979.

A good survey of the current state of health, especially alternative healing. Not as radical as many books from this group. Good text for a survey course.

Tubesing, Donald A. *Wholistic Health.* N.Y.: Human Sciences Press, 1978.

Tubesing describes the current dilemma of health care in compelling, human terms for both patient and provider. He then describes the approach taken in Wholistic Health Centers, and some challenges for the future. Some material is repeated from Wholistic Health Center monographs.

Tubesing, Nancy, et al. *Philosophical Assumptions of Wholistic Health Care.* Wholistic Health Centers, Inc., 1975.

Still one of the best expositions of the wholistic philosophy (unbiased opinion). Needs to be balanced by emphasis on health promotion and wellness.

Psychosomatics and Stress

Anderson, Robert A. *Stress Power!.* Human Sciences Press, 1978.

This Family Practice physician from the University of Washington can't be all bad, because he wears a bow tie. His book is readable and comprehensive. Too bad the publisher made it all look so superficial. A good text for a class in stress management, when it comes out in paperback. Excellent bibliography.

Cousins, Norman. *Anatomy of an Illness: Reflections on Healing and Regeneration.* N.Y.: Norton, 1979.

Cousins describes his own recovery from illness and reflects on subjects such as "Longevity and Creativity" and "Pain is not the ultimate enemy." Also includes physicians' responses to his experiences and ideas. Good bibliography. Compliments Pelletier's book.

Friedman, Meyer and Rosenman, Ray H. *Type A Behavior and Your Heart.* Knopf, 1974.

A hinge-point book in the relationship between behavior and heart disease. Much follow-up research has followed this work which clarifies and reinforces the findings. Not much help about changing in this book. Read together with Tillich's sermon, "You Are Accepted." (Type A's don't know Grace.)

Lynch, James J. *The Broken Heart: The Medical Consequences of Loneliness.* N.Y.: Basic Books, 1977.

Lynch gives verification to what the ancient Hebrews knew 3,000 years ago; that Exile and Death are the same word.

McQuade, Walter and Aikman, Ann. *Stress.* N.Y.: Bantam Books, 1974.

Guess what this book is about. A popularized expansion of a *Fortune* magazine article. Good for classes, and has a good summary of the Type A interview in the appendix.

Pelletier, Kenneth. *Mind as Healer, Mind as Slave.* N.Y.: Dell, 1977.

Pelletier is one of the leading figures in the "holistic" movement; an often outspoken advocate of self-care, especially emotional/physical relationships. His emphasis on the "mind's" regulation of health is very clear. A key book. Good bibliography of psychosomatic source material.

Selye, Hans. *Stress Without Distress.* N.Y.: Lippencott, 1974.

An essential book on stress by the physiologist who applied the term to human life in 1956 in *The Stress of Life.* He takes a shot at moral philosophy by re-writing the Golden Rule to be: "Earn your neighbor's love." As a theologian, he makes a better physiologist. A flood of other books on stress have followed, with clever titles such as *Stress, Stress!,* and *Stress Power!* We've discovered that it's okay to be under stress, but it's not okay to be nuts.

Tanner, Ogden, et al. *Stress, the Time-Life Book.* Time, Inc., 1976.

A Time-Life style look at the phenomenon of stress in a photojournalistic approach. Very interesting coverage of crisis, war and disaster relative to stress (sounds like family life). Not much talk about personal dynamics or what to do about it.

Self-Care and Wellness

Self-Care and Wellness
Ardell, Donald. *High Level Wellness.* Rodale Press, 1977.

Ardell is the focus of the wellness movement which encourages people to move beyond good health into greater levels of functioning. Short on spiritual dimensions, and on reasons why you should be so well, other than because it is there. Practical follow-up can be found in the *Wellness Workbook* by John W. Travis, available from Wellness Resource Center, Mill Valley, California 94941.

Benson, Herbert and Klipper, Miriam Z. *The Relaxation Response.* Avon, 1976.

A basic introduction to the physiology of relaxation and meditation, including some research results. Popular reading, and very simplistic about the actual practice of meditation. Good companion books are LeShan's *How To Meditate* and Kelsey's *The Other Side of Silence.*

Boston Women's Health Book Collective. *Our Bodies, Ourselves.* N.Y.: Simon & Schuster, 1971.

About ten years ago, the idea that women own their own bodies was radical feminism. It still is in many places, including much of health care. This is the women's health consciousness-raising classic, updated to include very good information on self-care.

Cooper, Kenneth. *The New Aerobics.* M. Evans, 1970.

The primary developer of the aerobic concept, Cooper (his center is in Texas) gives clear guidelines for the development of endurance fitness. Should be required reading for people planning to "get back in shape (puff, puff)."

Ferguson, James and Taylor, C. Barr. *A Change for Heart: Your Family and the Food You Eat.* Palo Alto, Calif.: Bull Publishing, 1978.

A family-oriented workbook full of charts and records for a seven week transition to a healthy diet. Could be fun for a group of families!

Ferguson, Tom, ed. *Medical Self-Care.* Box 717, Inverness, California 94937.

Periodic (about three per year) issues with well-written articles on exercise, self-examination, stress management, pharmaceuticals, etc. No advertising, so no vested interest in selling stuff. Highly recommended.

Great Waters of France, Inc. *The Perrier Study: Fitness in America.* 595 Madison Avenue, New York 10022.

An interesting and useful study by Louis Harris & Associates on the behaviors and attitudes of Americans toward physical fitness. Available free by writing the above address.

Johnson, G. Timothy, ed. *The Harvard Medical School Health Letter.* Cambridge, Mass.: Harvard University.

A monthly newsletter of health information, often paralleling current events or controversies, such as radiation hazards, immunization and saccharine. Good balance of professional and lay information.

Roberts, Toni M., et al. *Healthwise Handbook.*
Good companion to *Take Care of Yourself.* Excellent for young parents, because it includes guidance and encouragement for examination of children and self at home. Both books are strong foundation for a course in self-care.

Simonton, Carl, et al. *Getting Well Again: A Step-by-Step Guide to Overcoming Cancer.* Los Angeles, Calif.: J. P. Tarcher, Inc., 1978.
Describes Simonton's important work in cancer therapy which can be used as an adjunct to traditional treatment. Radical self-care and visualization are important elements.

Vickery, Donald M. and Fries, James R. *Take Care of Yourself.* Addison-Wesley, 1981.
A very useful set of protocols for decision-making about health problems. Tends to be conservative, encouraging you to check with the doctor more than you may feel necessary. Two relevant studies: when this book was used by one group, the physician contacts increased; when people were given the book and $50 for not calling the physician, the contacts decreased. Once more, economics rears its ugly head!

Westberg, Granger, E. *Good Grief.* Philadelphia: Fortress Press, 1962.
The classic in grief-as-a-healthy-process. Originally a sermon, this book can be read in an hour. And it's still inexpensive ($1.50). New edition has sexist language changed and a classy orange cover. Now available in large print editions. Compare with Lindemann's classic study: "Symptom Motology and Management of Acute Grief," in *Crisis Intervention,* by Parad, 1973.

Wurtman, Judith. *Eating Your Way Through Life.* N.Y.: Raven Press, 1979.
There are literally hundreds of nutrition books out, and this is one of the best. Wurtman is readable and informative. She's a

Ph.D. on the staff of M.I.T., and regularly teaches health professionals. Use this hard-to-get book for nutrition classes.

Compiled by William M. Peterson, M.Div.ACSW
Wholistic Health Centers, Inc.
137 Smith Garfield Street
Hinsdale, Il. 60521

Acknowledgments

Many people have encouraged me in the preparation of this book. Thanks go to Cheryl Forbes and Judith Markham of Zondervan for their interest in the project and especially for Judith's skillful refinement of the manuscript. Thanks to Sharon Murfin of Missoula, Montana, who spent many tedious hours typing the manuscript and its subsequent revisions, for the confidence she expressed in me during the process.

From the day I first received the telephone call encouraging me to write this book, my husband Wes has been a constant partner in the project. He has generously given both his own editorial skills and, more costly still, his commitment to co-parenting our son JonKrister so that I could enjoy uninterrupted blocks of time with the manuscript.

The origins of this book, however, began while I was a student at Wesley Theological Seminary in Washington, D.C. where, under the direction of Dr. Charles W. Stewart, professor of pastoral psychology, I wrote my religious life history, several case histories, and finally my thesis on healing and the church. These writing experiences were foundational to my choosing to focus on the whole person—particularly on the role of a person's faith in the healing process.

I have also been profoundly affected by my relationship with three unique church communities: the Church of the Saviour, Washington, D.C., Sojourners Fellowship, Washington, D.C., and Community Covenant Church, Missoula, Montana. In these three churches, I have experienced most directly what it means for people to strive for wholeness in body, mind, and spirit. I cannot speak boldly enough about the healing power present in Christ's gathered Body. But the woman I have called Helene has done just that in the offering of her story. Knowing her and being free to share her story added an unexpected depth to the case for treating the whole person.

-KGM-